Childhood Obesity: A Biobehavioral Perspective

Childhood Obesity

A Biobehavioral Perspective

Edited by

Norman A. Krasnegor, Ph.D.

Human Learning and Behavior Branch
Center for Research for Mothers and Children
National Institute of Child Health and Human Development
National Institutes of Health
Bethesda, Maryland

Gilman D. Grave, M.D.

Endocrinology, Nutrition and Growth Branch
Center for Research for Mothers and Children
National Institute of Child Health and Human Development
National Institutes of Health
Bethesda, Maryland

Norman Kretchmer, M.D., Ph.D.

Department of Nutritional Sciences
University of California, Berkeley
Department of Pediatrics and Obstetrics
University of California, San Francisco

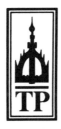

THE TELFORD PRESS
Caldwell, New Jersey

THE TELFORD PRESS, INC.
285 Bloomfield Avenue, Caldwell, New Jersey, 07006

Library of Congress Cataloging-in-Publication Data

Childhood obesity: a biobehavioral perspective/edited by Norman A.
  Krasnegor, Gilman D. Grave, Norman Kretchmer.
      p.   cm.
    Includes bibliographies and index.
    ISBN 0-936923-05-9: $45.00. ISBN 0-936923-04-0 (pbk.): $25.50
    1. Obesity in children. I. Krasnegor, Norman A. II. Grave;
  Gilman D., 1941– . III. Kretchmer, Norman, 1923– .
    [DNLM: 1. Obesity — in infancy & childhood. 2. Obesity-prevention
  & control.   WD 210 C5373]
  RJ399.C6C473 1988
  618.92′398 — dc 19
  DNLM/DLC

Contents

Preface

NORMAN A. KRASNEGOR and GILMAN D. GRAVE
National Institute of Child
Health and Human Development
National Institutes of Health
Bethesda, Maryland

Epidemiological data, based upon studies of adults, strongly implicate obesity as a significant risk factor for hypertension, atherosclerotic cardio-vascular disease, and type II diabetes mellitus. The prevention of obesity should therefore be of the highest priority on the agenda for the public health. Given such a goal, a rational strategy is to determine when and under what conditions obesity is first manifested. Many scientists and clinicians have therefore focused their research upon discovering the necessary and sufficient conditions which foster the emergence of obesity in childhood. A clear understanding of the behavioral and biological factors of etiological relevence during this phase of development can be instrumental in promoting health and establishing effective treatments.

Evidence derived from the Health and Nutrition Examination Surveys (HANES) collected by the National Center for Health Statistics reveals that the prevalence of obesity among children is increasing. For example, William Dietz (this volume) has determined that obesity prevalence has increased 54% among 6–11 year olds and 39% among teenagers (12–17 year olds) during the past two decades. Others have shown that obesity tracks from age four and the risk for adult obesity increases with age thereafter. These findings reinforce the importance of studying obesity within a developmental context.

This volume highlights recent research findings which elucidate the biological and behavioral underpinnings of childhood obesity. The book is divided into four sections: Perspectives, Determinants, Prevention and Treatment.

1. Perspectives

This section includes two chapters. The first of these is written by Norman Kretchmer, a co-editor of this work and well-known researcher in the field of pediatric nutrition. In his essay on the topic he asks the question: What is obesity? Whereas it is clear that there is no direct answer to this question, his chapter poses a number of issues for researchers who study the topic. A major thrust of his essay is that a biopsychosocial approach provides a necessary research framework to gain a meaningful perspective on what obesity is and the health consequences that it poses for children.

Lisa Buckmaster and Kelly Brownell provide the reader with a look at the social and psychological factors that comprise the obese child's world in the second chapter of this section. The authors provide an appreciation for the social environment and its power to affect the lives of children. They summarize important research findings concerning the role of family, self-concept, peer behavior, and social support in the development and management of obesity. A central conclusion of their findings is that, for many people who are obese, the psychological and social consequences may outweigh the medical implications.

II. Determinants

The section on determinants contains five chapters. Roger Siervogel's manuscript on genetic and familial factors that affect obesity reviews in meticulous detail the approaches used in the past for studying this question. He reviews the evidence which links familial factors to the likelihood of becoming obese. His chapter includes a superb guide to employing a genetic-epidemiological approach for conducting research. This narrative provides the reader with a clear understanding of the methodological approach, its value in framing questions, and a way to untangle the hard nature/nurture issues posed by childhood obesity.

Siervogel's work is followed by that of W. Stewart Agras. His chapter focuses upon the question of whether eating patterns early in life influence adiposity later in development. The research he summarizes suggests that there is a relationship between caloric intake and adiposity in infancy. He clearly outlines for the reader the three lines of evidence. These include: (a) studies of relationships between energy intake and adiposity; (b) rate of weight gain and later adiposity; (c) mode of feeding and adiposity. His summary of studies on infant feeding and adiposity should be included on the syllabus of any student of this topic.

The next chapter is by David L. Margules. In his essay he describes two types of opioid peptides, their respective receptor sites, and effects they produce when released. He hypothesizes that peptides which occupy epsilon-mu receptors when released produce stupefaction and are associated with being overweight. Those opioids which occupy delta receptors in the brain are associated with hyperactivity and lean body mass. He describes a series of hypotheses concerning the role of beta-endorphin and serotonin in the initiation and maintenance of obesity. He also describes his experiments which implicate enkephalin analogues in the initiation of migration-like running. His chapter offers an intriguing set of ideas concerning the causation of obesity and new ways to think about treating it.

Paul Rozin's chapter, which follows, examines the question of putative relationships between food preferences and obesity. His work provides the reader with a critical analysis of what is meant by food preference and how researchers distinguish between preference and liking. He analyzes what has been learned by scientists about the mechanisms which underpin the acquisition of food preference. Further, he reviews what has been learned and hypothesized about links between obesity and food preference.

In the final chapter of this section, Robert C. Klesges provides a combined overview of methodological and integration issues that confront researchers who study childhood obesity. Regarding methodology he reviews the pertinent literature and problems associated with how to measure dietary intake and physical activity. He also presents a thoughtful discussion of the multisystemic nature of obesity. This latter recognition strongly suggests that "the" cause of obesity does not exist. Obesity is conceptualized as being multidetermined. This perspective argues that a deep understanding of childhood obesity can only be attained by studying the child, his/her family and peers.

III. Prevention

The third section of the book includes two chapters that focus upon prevention. The first of these is contributed by Debra G. Clark and Steven N. Blair. The main focus of their work addresses the issue of whether inactivity causes and/or exacerbates obesity. The authors point to the increased risk for adult obesity if an individual is obese as a child. They point out that research on the relationship between physical activity and obesity in childhood is meager. They report on recent developments which the Institute for Aerobics Research has undertaken to standardize reporting of physical activity. The Fitnessgram is a computerized system for assessing and reporting physical fitness levels of school children (grades K–12). The data from their sample suggests a strong relationship between physical fitness, physical activity and adiposity. They feel that it is premature to conclude that a causal relationship exists between a sedentary lifestyle and obesity in children and youth.

The chapter by Guy S. Parcel, Lawrence W. Green and Barbara S. Bettes examines the experience to date in designing and implementing school based programs to prevent obesity in school children. One generalization that emerges from their review of the extant literature on intervention is that the most effective approaches require that children and their parents be involved in treatment (see also Israel and Epstein this volume). A second finding discussed by the authors is that interventions which involve lifestyle changes in physical activity coupled with behavior modification have a greater likelihood for success in treating obese children. They indicate that school-based programs which target energy input and expenditure are the most likely to be successful for the greatest percentage of children considered overweight. Another significant variable for school-based programs is the age of the participants. Children in elementary school appear to be more successful at weight control programs than junior high school students. The authors also introduce a note of caution regarding the potential of intervention programs to cause harm in the form of labeling, coercion and excessive food restriction.

IV.   Treatment

This section of the book contains four chapters. The first, authored by Sue Y.S. Kimm, gives an overview of the necessary concerns involved in the provision of quality medical care to the obese child and his/her family. She advocates the use of careful medical history and growth charts to help establish the proper diagnosis. In addition, she cautions that thorough examinations should evaluate the morbidity associated with obesity. The author points out that several levels of psychosocial evaluation should be undertaken with an obese child. She also points out that the nature of complaints associated with the obesity can be helpful in assessing parental motivation. Kimm argues that the physician should evaluate the child's motivation and perception of his/her weight status. The author points out that effective treatment implies good measures of change in adiposity. She advocates the use of skinfold calipers and waist measurement as adjuncts to body weight. She also reviews safety issues concerning dietary restrictions in the growing child.

Kimm's chapter is followed by that of William H. Dietz, whose work focuses upon metabolic factors involved in dieting. He provides an excellent overview of methodological problems inherent in the design of studies to evaluate the effects of hypocaloric diets on obese patients. His chapter provides a critical analysis of research on the interrelationships among nitrogen balance, protein and glucose metabolism. He also discusses fat loss and concludes that it remains unclear which diet is optimal for maximizing fat loss. Dietz also highlights behavioral problems associated with adherence as being an essential key to weight reduction. Along with other contributors to this volume, he, too, emphasizes the importance of family dynamics in the design of effective treatment programs for obese children.

The chapter by Allen Israel echoes the views of Klesges (this volume) concerning the necessary role of parental and family influences in childhood obesity. He views these influences as central to gaining a meaningful understanding of what obesity is and how to treat it effectively in children. Israel argues that parents must attend and participate in the treatment sessions of their obese child. Along with parental weight loss as a strategy for involvement, he suggests that the parent act in the role of helper. He also points to the value of enhancing parenting skills through training to implement child behavior change. Finally, he provides an overview of family variables which may help identify particular populations that ought to be targeted for prevention or early interventions.

In the final chapter in this section, Leonard H. Epstein provides a selective review of research on treatment intervention. Epstein points out that without intervention many obese children become obese adults. Therefore interventions during childhood might serve well to prevent adult obesity and the morbidity associated with it. The family-based program of research discussed by the author focuses upon changing eating and exercises behaviors. Epstein found a strong relationship in his treatment intervention research program between parent and child weight loss. What is significant about the research reviewed is that it is based upon a longitudinal design that was conducted over a five-year period. While parental involvement is seen as important for treatment success, Epstein also implicates the relevance of self-control factors in weight-loss programs. He also reviews evidence to date on exercise. Lifestyle related exercise was found to be superior to high intensity aerobic exercise for reducing weight. However, adherence to an exercise regimen is a problem for obese children. This factor must therefore be taken into consideration when designing an exercise program for overweight children.

This volume provides a needed addition to the literature on childhood obesity. Its framework, predicated upon a biobehavioral perspective of this major public health problem, will be of significant benefit to students, researchers, and clinicians who have an interest in interdisciplinary research. The book will, we hope, become a standard reference for workers in the fields of behavioral pediatrics, behavioral medicine and public health.

I

PERSPECTIVES

1

Introduction:
What is Obesity

NORMAN KRETCHMER
Department of Nutritional Sciences
University of California, Berkeley
Department of Pediatrics and Obstetrics
University of California, San Francisco

During the past three decades there have been considerable advances in our understanding of the complex mechanisms involved in the production of obesity. The authors in this volume have made major advances in the area of childhood obesity. I have been reviewing the literature on obesity for some time and have found it necessary to resort to review articles because it is impossible to absorb the vast amount of material in the literature. And it is difficult to separate good from bad.

Obesity is a complex biological situation and a prime example of a problem where there is constant interaction of genetics and environment. It is fruitless to argue which of these components, genetics or environment, nature or nurture, has more significance in the production of obesity. I think there are good examples at both ends of the spectrum. There is a clear genetic example in the mouse, particularly in the yellow mouse. However, yellow mice can be thin *or* fat depending upon whether the animals are active or not. In the human there are the examples of the Pima Papago Indians of Phoenix, or the Samoans who are often obese as a result of eating large amounts of poor food and refined carbohydrates. The complexities of appetite can be enumerated by starting with sensory aspects and ending with satiety. Both physiologic features require neurological and hormonal stimuli. Two years ago a Consensus Conference on Obesity was held at the NIH (Foster and Burton, 1985). The major question that emerged was: What is obesity? This is a very difficult question to answer, for there are many different opinions, some based on culture and others on science. The definition of obesity has changed over the years, and what we would call obesity today would not have been discerned as obesity yesterday.

In the technical sense, medical personnel have considerable difficulty defining obesity and often take the easy path by defining individuals as obese when they are 120% or more of their ideal weight. Similarly, individuals who are 150% or more of their ideal weight are said to be truly obese, and those who are twice or more than their ideal weight are said to have malignant obesity. But, weight is not necessarily a good measure of obesity. For example, a big person who weighs a great deal may be more lean than he or she is fat. It is unreasonable to call such an individual obese.

In nutritional science this problem is approached by using arithmetic formulas that remove the idiosyncrasies of weight and height. One such function is body mass index, which is defined as weight in kilograms divided by height in meters squared. A body mass index of 27.8 is considered by some authors to separate normal from obese males. However, body mass index is not sufficiently descriptive because there is no consideration of lean body mass. Garn, Clark and Guire (1975) use skinfolds to estimate fat. Skinfold measurements to estimate fat are reasonable measures when used for adults but are a poor measurement of fat in children, and they are replete with error when used in infants. Such measurements are fraught with gross inter-observer errors.

Dr. William Weil (1981) of Michigan State University wrote a very interesting article some years ago. In it he outlined perceptions of obesity made by an involved child and by significant other people in the child's environment. He said one could consider obesity as an illness, and that an obese person is disgusting. Is this an apt definition? Does a child think of obesity as an illness? Suppose that one thinks of obesity as an illness, or as a disability, either physical, mental or social. Note that some teachers think obesity may reflect a mental disability. Regarding the social disability definition of obesity, a child may find that he is somewhat impaired in his activity. Is obesity a defect without dysfunction? Everybody seems to think so, according to Weil. With mild dysfunction? With severe dysfunction? Is obesity a medical risk factor? Physicians argue that individuals who are more than 120% of their ideal weight are certainly obese, and that those who are 150% or more of their ideal body weight are definitely at increased risk in terms of illnesses that might develop later in life.

There has been much conjecture about the etiology of obesity. A simplistic theorem suggests that, if energy in exceeds energy out, one will gain weight. Researchers have pointed out, though, that energy utilized has many biological antecedents. Thus, for example, an Eskimo living in a cold climate depends on thermogenesis to maintain body temperature.

The Eskimo under these conditions can ingest considerable amounts of energy-containing food and not gain weight. Scott and Amundsen in their quest for the South Pole ate about 6,000 calories a day; but they lost weight. In fact, Scott died of starvation, scurvy and a variety of other nutritional problems.

So, a discussion of energy balance must consider activity, endogenous metabolism, absorption of energy, thermogenesis and the efficient use of energy. Forbes (1984) recalculated data gathered by a physiologist named Neumann (1902) and by Gulick (1922). These two men increased their weight in the range of about 50 to 90 grams a day when they exceeded their required caloric needs. Each was different in size, and one was more athletic than the other. Gulick was younger than Neumann. Their body mass indices differed: Gulick's was 20, while Neumann's was 24. They were both below the commonly accepted body mass index designating obesity. Weight for both increased or decreased if the intake of calories fluctuated. The energy equivalent of weight change for Neumann was 9.2 kcal/g, and that for Gulick 7.2 kcal/g. As the data indicate, a small steady increase in caloric intake could lead to a substantial increase in weight over a period of a year. Since most people seem to remain within 10% of the weight they attained by age 25, there appears to be a setpoint for weight.

Fat is contained in specialized cells, the adipocytes. They, as all cells, go through the process of proliferation and maturation. In the former case there is an increase in cell number and in the latter, cell size. In a population of cells both proliferation and maturation occur, often simultaneously. It is only by observing a single cell that both processes can be separated.

Obesity is typified by larger cells — hypertropic cells replete with stored fat. Although the adipocytes increase in the nonobese individual, the number of adipose cells increases remarkably in the obese individual. Also, it appears that adipocytes from a fat person do not release fat as easily as do adipocytes from a thin person, or a lean person when the tissue is stimulated with epinephrine (Knittle et al. 1981). Even after reduction in weight, there is a tendency for the cells to retain the fat in the fat cells of the originally obese person. The intricate mechanisms of this phenomenon have to be studied.

Genetic factors have also been demonstrated to contribute to the etiology of obesity (see Siervogel in this volume). If an individual has two obese parents, the odds of his or her becoming obese are high (Garn and Clark 1976). If one has two lean parents the likelihood of staying lean is excellent while mixtures of lean and obese parents produce more complex outcomes. Data presented by Stunkard et al. (1986), for example, show that twins born to obese parents and subsequently placed with lean adoptive parents will have a higher probability of being obese than not. These observations need careful consideration.

Other factors also influence the likelihood of becoming obese. Thus, color, odor, and taste preferences are important influences on people's eating behavior and appetite. For example, if red dye were removed from hot dogs, few people would eat the resulting gray dogs. Olfactory and gustatory cues are important for eating behavior. From an anecdotal perspective it is clear that odor is important. For example, if one walks into a delicatessen and smells its distinctive odor, a usual response is salivation.

I would like to review the data that derived from the NIH Consensus Conference (Foster and Burton, 1985). The first problem is that the percent of males overweight by race and age show practically no difference. However, there is a large racial difference in females. For overweight non-pregnant females at all ages, the black female tends to be heavier. In our clinic, 80% of the black teengers encountered are more than 120% above ideal weight. The explanations for these findings are cuisine and lack of activity. However, none of the explanations are satisfactorily documented epidemiologically. The percent of non- pregnant females overweight by poverty status and age indicate that the poverty groups tend to be heavier. Of the Hispanic group of patients at the San Francisco General Hospital, 25% are 120% above ideal weight. Consequently, we have a very high rate of gestational diabetes. I am sure that other hospitals with a similar patient population would have the same statistics. Males in the poverty group are usually not overweight.

There are a number of statements in the literature describing the personality traits and the biobehavioral problems of obese children and teenagers (Peck and Ullrich, 1985). Some of these declarations are difcult to deal with and others seem to be very practical. Are there specific behavioral characteristics that predict obesity, or that are associated with obesity? Social contacts also exert a considerable psychological pressure on the obese individual and all of these behavioral considerations compound the complexity of obesity.

The relationship of physical disease to obesity is an area of great interest. For example, an obese individual is more likely to have ischemic heart disease in the presence of other factors, such as hypertension, diabetes, inactivity, smoking, elevated triglycerides and elevated LDL cholesterol. In these cases obesity increases the risks considerably. But, if there are none of those complications in an individual who is overweight, then there is no greater risk of ischemic cardiac disease than in an individual of normal weight.

The occurrence of diabetes with obesity is more likely. This kind of diabetes can be called adult-onset and maturity-onset diabetes or a type of Type II diabetes mellitus. In certain ethnic groups it is a post-receptor diabetes, associated with hyperinsulinism.

We can identify three issues that reflect our concern with the current attitude toward children and how their growth and development are perceived in relation to weight. These issues are: 1) our society is overly concerned about body size and conformation to a slim image, 2) individual needs of the child are not adequately considered, and 3) in current health practices interventions are sometimes overly aggressive and focus on a single aspect of the problem, usually the diet. These issues imply a need for research into cost benefit studies of prevention, parenting processes, therapy of disturbed eating habits, identification of risks of obesity, and research into energy metabolism.

A set of questions on the health implications of obesity were considered by the Consensus Group that met at NIH in 1985. They wanted to know, as I would: What is obesity? What is the evidence that obesity has adverse effects on health? What is the evidence that obesity affects longevity? What are the appropriate uses and limitations of existing height/weight tables? For what medical conditions should weight reduction be recommended? What should be the direction of future research in this area? They suggested as future research, the search for biological markers in infancy and childhood so that a prediction can be made as to whether an individual would be at risk for obesity.

My conclusions are as follows: Obesity is an incredibly complex problem. Obesity is in part determined by our cultural and socioeconomic environment. At the moment our culture says, "You dare not be obese." This statement is made for a variety of reasons. We do not like it. You do not look good. It may affect your health. I think it is going to take the combined effort of biobehavioral scientists who deal with aspects of obesity as well as physiologic scientists to define clearly the biological complexities involved in obesity. I expect that the following contributions in this volume will be enlightening.

References

Bray, G. A. (1986). Adolescent obesity. In: *Frontiers in Clinical Nutrition* N. Kretchmer (Ed.). Aspen Systems Corporation. Rockville, MD: pp. 153–183.

Forbes, G. B. (1984). Energy intake and body weight: A reexamination of two "classic" studies. *Am. J. Clin. Nutr. 39*:349–350.

Foster, W. R. & Burton B. T. (Eds.). (1985). Health implications of obesity, Part 2. National Institutes of Health Consensus Development Conference. *Ann. Int. Med. 103*: 979–1077.

Garn, S. M. & Clark, D. C. (1976). Trends in fatness and origins of obesity. *Pediatrics, 57*: 443–456.

Garn, S. M., Clark, D. C. & Guire, K. E. (1975). Growth, body composition, and development of obese and lean children. In *Childhood Obesity* (pp. 23–46). New York, John Wiley. M. Winick (Ed)

Gulick, A. (1922). A Study of weight regulation in the adult human body during overnutrition. *Am. J. Physiol. 60*:371–395.

Knittle, J. L., Merritt, R. J., Dixon-Shanies, D., Ginsberg-Fellner, F., Timmers, K. I. & Katz, D. P. (1981). Childhood obesity. In R. M. Suskind (Ed.), *Textbook of Pediatric Nutrition*, pp. 415–434. New York: Raven Press.

Neumann, R. O. (1902). Experimentelle Beitrage zur Lehre von dem taglichen Nahrungsbedarf des Menschen unter besonderer Berucksichtigung der notwendigen Eiweissmenge. *Arch. Hyg. 45*:1–87.

Peck, E. B. & Ullrich, H. (1985). *Children and Weight: A Changing Perspective.* pp. 1–29. Berkeley, CA: Nutrition Communications Associates.

Stunkard, A. J., Sorensen, T. I. A., Hanis, C., Teasdale, T. W., Chakraborty, R., Schull, W. J. & Schulsinger, F. (1986). An adoption study of human obesity. *New Eng. J. Med. 314*:193–198.

Weil, W. B., Jr. (1981). Obesity: a problem in perceptions. In *Infant and Child Feeding* pp. 333–342. Bellflower, CA: Academic Press, Inc.

2

The Social and Psychological World of the Obese Child

LISA BUCKMASTER
Department of Psychology
Willamette University
Salem, Oregon

KELLY D. BROWNELL
Department of Psychiatry
University of Pennsylvania
Philadelphia, Pennsylvania

The goal of this chapter is to provide the reader with an appreciation for the power of the social environment in influencing childhood obesity. We will first review the literature which has examined the social climate of the obese child. Then, the concept of social support will be discussed along with its relationship to health and wellness. Finally, approaches to treatment and prevention incorporating social support will be addressed and implications for future directions will be suggested. Understanding the social world of the obese child is necessary to develop a comprehensive, biobehavioral perspective on childhood obesity.

I. The Social and Psychological Climate of the Obese Child

In examining the world of obese children, we must look at peers, family, schools, socioeconomic class, and genetics. Additionally, it is important to determine how they interact with their physical environment, that is, how active or passive they are in day-to-day life. Let us consider what the obese child encounters as a result of his or her weight.

The social and psychological effects of obesity can be difficult for children (Brownell, 1982; Stunkard, 1976; Brownell and Stunkard, 1978; Israel and Shapiro, 1985). The major problem is not the excess weight alone, but the view of others in the social environment. Obese children are often the target of ridicule. They are teased, excluded from peer groups, and picked last for athletic activities. Obese children will seek excuses to avoid gym class because of intense shame of their bodies (Brownell, 1984).

The pervasive bias against obesity is exhibited by children as young as six years of age. Obese children are rated by six-year-olds as less likeable than children with a variety of physical handicaps, and children attribute to a picture of a fat child they do not know characteristics such as "lazy, sloppy, devious, absentminded, dirty, and stupid" (Maddox, Back, and Liederman, 1968; Staffieri, 1967). Furthermore, children believe that obese children are to blame for their corpulence and that the obesity results solely from excessive self-indulgence (Edelman, 1982). Canning and Mayer (1966) found that overweight high school students were less likely to be admitted to high ranking colleges than were their thin peers, even when controlling for grades and extracurricular activities. As adolescents, obese children may be less likely to date and more likely to be withdrawn (Brownell, 1986).

Whether the discriminatory treatment of the obese child by peers results in negative psychologial sequelae is controversial. While clinical observations suggest that obese children experience low self-esteem as a result of their weight (Allon, 1979), objective studies have demonstrated contradictory findings. Sallade's (1973) study indicated that obese children had significantly lower self-esteem than did their normal-weight peers as measured by the Piers-Harris Children's Self-Concept Scale. Using the same instrument, Mendelson and White (1982) and Wadden, Foster, Brownell, and Finley (1984) did not detect differences between obese and non-obese children in self-esteem.

Two aspects of this research are puzzling. First is the discrepancy among studies using the same scale (Piers-Harris Self-Concept Scale), but this is common in social science research. Second is the dichotomy between intuition and clinical experience on the one hand and research on the other. If one asks health professionals, educators, fat people and thin people, there is general agreement that obesity is a social disadvantage which influences psychological functioning, including self-concept. We can dismiss intuition in favor of published studies, can dismiss the studies, or can accept both intuition and research and presume that studies have not yet tapped the area of psychological functioning influenced by life experiences as an obese person. We feel this last stance is most likely to yield valuable information.

Self-concept scales may not be sensitive to the subtleties of the long- and short-term effects of discriminatory practices among children and society toward the obese child. It must be asked, "Do these instruments measure what we need to measure?" Global measures may not identify the critical variables in assessing the psychological impact on the obese child. One recent study found that global measures of assertion, depression, and self-consciousness did not differentiate obese from lean subjects (Klesges, 1984). However, when specific items regarding weight were involved, marked differences were evident (Klesges, 1984; Mendelson and White, 1985). Would another self-image questionnaire yield different results? Additionally, behavioral indices regarding rate and type of social interactions of obese children and non-obese children would help clarify whether differences exist at a more overt level. Behaviorally, it has been demonstrated that obese adolescent girls are often withdrawn, passive and isolated in response to peer discrimination (Monello and Mayer, 1963).

While no differences between obese and non-obese children have been found in psychological disturbance or psychopathology when seen for medical procedures (Wadden and Stunkard, 1985), weight specific problems may still be influential. Complications likely to affect the quality of life without affecting scores on psychological tests are lack of confidence due to the inability to maintain weight loss and a sense of isolation when family, friends and physicians cannot understand the frustrations of the weight problem.

Apart from the psychological manifestations of obesity, other cultural, biological and environmental influences have a direct impact upon the obese child's world. The best predictor of childhood obesity in the United States is the socioeconomic class an individual is born into (Stunkard, 1975). The incidence of obesity is highest in the lower socioeconomic groups and lowest in the upper socioeconomic groups in the American culture. Into adulthood, SES is the single best predictor of weight for females. The pressure for women to conform to svelte stereotypes is pronounced in some subcultures, while obesity is accepted in others. This creates wide differences in eating practices, the frequency of dieting, and body image.

Certainly, social factors are not the only factors influencing obesity. Genetics appear to play a pronounced role. In a demographic study of adopted children, weights of the natural parents directly correlated with the offspring's adult weights, even though the children were raised by adoptive parents whose weights did not correlate with their adopted children's weight (Stunkard et al., 1986). It is not possible to identify cause and effect relationships here because a number of factors covary with both weight and demographics. Clearly, genetics and the environment are operating to affect the child's weight. This study would suggest a genetic predisposition toward slimness or obesity. We must look at what environmental factors can influence such a predisposition.

II. Behavioral Aspects of Childhood Obesity

What occurs in the everyday life of the obese child to affect his or her weight? What effects do parents, peers and the environment have in determining food intake and activity level, the two major behavioral components in the energy balance equation? If we pursue this question in keeping with social learning theory, we must examine stimulus, reinforcement and cognitive variables.

There are at least two types of stimulus control which influence childhood eating patterns. The first consists simply of the availability and familiarity of food in the environment. Children's familiarity with food accounts for 25 to 30% of the variability in their food preferences (Birch, 1979 (a), 1979 (b)). The influence of familiarity is equivalent to that of sweetness (Birch, 1979 (a), 1979 (b)). The power of food familiarity was best demonstrated by Birch and Marlin, who exposed children to novel cheeses and fruits (Birch and Marlin, 1982). They found a linear relationship between the amount of exposure and preference. This implies that children will prefer what they are exposed to at home. Similarly, children show aversions for foods their parents do not like (McCarthy, 1935).

Peer and parental prompting may also serve as stimuli to childhood eating. Klesges and his associates (Klesges, Malott, Boschee, and Weber 1986; Klesges, et al. 1983) demonstrated that relative weight in two-year-olds correlated positively with parental prompts to eat. Parents of obese children prompted 2.3 times as much eating as parents of normal weight children.

Parental encouragement of physical activity follows similar patterns. Parental prompting to be active is significantly correlated with child activity (Klesges et al., 1986; Klesges et al., 1984). Children in these studies who were more active had lower relative weights. Parental promotion to be active correlated negatively with the childrens' relative weight.

Children appear to prefer foods that parents use as reinforcers. Birch, Zimmerman and Hind (1980) demonstrated that children will change their preferences for foods that are used as reinforcers or foods associated with parental attention. Likewise, a school program using token econo-mies to encourage nutritionally balanced eating in five- and six-year-old obese children was effective in increasing consumption of nutritious snacks (Epstein, Masek and Marshall, 1978; Stark et al, 1986). Generali-zation of improved food choices to the home did not occur until the children were trained to cue their parents to praise new food choices.

Reinforcement can also influence physical activity. Epstein et al. (1984) found that physical activity in obese five-to-eight-year-old girls could be significantly modified by reinforcing active movement. The end result of the reinforcement was an increase in caloric expenditure of 40%.

Parental belief systems, or cognitive factors, also play an important role in childrens' eating. For example, parents often believe that children dislike skim milk, and that the temperature of milk will influence con-sumption. However, when children were presented with milk of varying fat density at different temperatures, no differences in consumption were noted (Herbert-Jackson, Cross and Risley, 1977). Perhaps because some parents dislike skim milk, they assume that their children do not like it. Similarly, sugar and salt added to baby foods may be for the parents' taste preferences, in the belief that the childrens' are the same (Foman, 1974).

Furthermore, parents' expectations influence not only what the child will eat, but the quantity of intake as well. Waxman and Stunkard (1980) revealed that parental beliefs affect obese childrens' consumption and level of physical activity. Believing that obese children "need" more to eat, parents will feed them more than their lean siblings. Likewise, parents expect the activity level of their obese children to be lower than that of their thin siblings. This expectation is shown from time-sampled activity assessments in the Waxman and Stunkard study. Obese boys were far less active than their thin controls inside the home, but only slightly less active outside the home and equally active at school.

Finally, modeling of peers, parents, and authority figures may serve as an important mediator in determining habit development in children's eating and activity level. Peer modeling can effect food selection (Birch, 1980; Marinho, 1942; Perry, Le Bow and Buser, 1979). Peer modeling has its most powerful impact on children who have not developed strong preferences for the foods being studied. In evaluating children's modeling of adults, Harper and Sanders (1975) compared the effects of prompts and modeling on children ranging in age from one to four. Children followed the adult model's eating behavior in 80% of the cases. However, when prompted to eat, children would respond only 48% of the time. While prompts to eat do influence intake, an adult model is even more powerful as a stimulus. Harper and Sanders' study used adult models who were unknown to the children. Therefore, studies must be done on parental prompts and modeling.

Beyond human interaction and its effect on eating, our environment is altered by technology that at times may substitute for human interaction. Watching television is one of the best examples of this point. Thus, Deitz and Gortmaker (1985) found that the prevalence of obesity increased by 2% for each additional hour of television viewed per day by 12- to 17-year-old adolescents. These authors were careful to control for prior obesity, geographic region, season, race, socioeconomic class, population density and a number of family variables. This suggests that television viewing may contribute to obesity in children. Such a hypothesis would be consistent with the effect of increased television viewing on physical activity and consumption of calorically dense foods. Besides the fact that television contributes to a more sedentary life-style, modeling of television characters' eating habits could also influence children's food choices. Advertisers are quick to take advantage of this phenomenon. It is likely that children increase their eating while they are watching television, and they eat more of the foods advertised on television (Kolata, 1986).

The picture of the obese child's world is colored by a combination of factors. There is likely to be a family predisposition toward obesity and modeling of family food choices. Additionally, peers will influence the child's eating behavior. They will make determinations regarding the obese child's social desirability. The presence of television in the child's world creates an environment geared to minimize physical activity, increase consumption, influence food choices, and decrease social interaction. Whereas social factors may be strong, they can be changed. It seems logical to suspect that the vehicle for modifying the effects of social factors would be via social support and manipulation of the child's social environment. Before examining how social support has been used in treating obese children, let us survey social support and its relationship to health and wellness.

III.   The Influence of Social Support Factors on Health

In the last fifteen years, there has been a dramatic surge of interest in the concept of social support as it pertains to health and well-being. This can be attributed to several factors. One factor is the increased awareness of the role of the social environment in the etiology of disease and illness. Another factor is the realization that social support may play a role in treatment. A third reason is that the concept of social support aids in the integration of the diverse literature on psychosocial factors and disease (Cohen and Syme, 1985).

Social support has been defined by Cohen and Syme (1985) as "the resources provided by other persons." Sarason, Levine, Basham and Sarason (1983) define social support as the "existence or availability of people on whom we can rely, people who let us know that they care about, value, and love us." Social support is generally broken down into four types: instrumental, emotional, informational and social companionship (Cohen and Wills, 1985). Instrumental support refers to the function of providing material support, for example, food, clothing, transportation, shelter, and financial assistance. Emotional support refers to the availability of those who can provide encouragement, constructive feedback and an outlet for emotional expression. Informational support comprises access to information regarding resources for an individual in order to optimize options, for example, what treatment programs are available, job openings, classes, etc. Finally, social companionship is spending time with others in recreational or leisure pursuits. There are several ways these functions mitigate the effects of stressful events and contribute to improved health.

There is a growing body of literature that links social support to health. The evidence of an association between social support and mental health and mortality is strong. However, the relationship between social support and physical illness is more controversial. While the mechanism linking social support to health is in dispute, two major theories have been posited.

The first of these theories is called the direct or main effect hypothesis. This suggests that positive relationships between social support and health occur because access to social support enhances health regardless of stress level. That is, the more social support one has whether under stress or not, the healthier that individual will be when compared to someone who has less social support. Supporting evidence occurs for the direct effect model regarding major health outcomes when contrasting persons who have very few or no social contacts to those who have a moderate or high level of "embeddedness" in social roles. In essence, beneficial effects of social support occur because larger social networks provide individuals with regular positive experiences, stable and predictable roles in the community, and a recognition of self-worth. Numerous studies demonstrate that people with spouses, friends, and family members who provide psychological and material resources are in better health than those with fewer supportive social contacts (Broadhead et al., 1983; Leavy, 1983; Mitchell, Billings, and Moos, 1982). In general it can be said that a lack of *positive* social relationships leads to negative psychological states. In turn, these psychological states may eventually impinge on physical health either through a direct effect on physiological processes which influence one's susceptibility to disease or through behavioral patterns (e.g., smoking, overeating, drinking, decreased activity level) that increase risk for disease and mortality.

The buffering hypothesis, on the other hand, proposes that social support protects people from potentially adverse effects of stressful events and serves as a resource to draw upon in times of trouble. If an individual appraises an event as stressful, feelings of helplessness may result. Given the nature of the stressful situation at hand, the appropriate kinds of support (i.e., informational, social companionship, emotional, and/or instrumental) can intercede to assuage the perceived threat of danger before the stressful event is totally disruptive (Cohen and Wills, 1985).

In a careful review of the literature on social support, Cohen and Wills (1985) conclude that there is evidence bolstering both models. The buffering model was found to operate when the social support measures assessed the perceived availability of interpersonal resources that were responsive to the needs elicited by stressful events. The direct effect hypothesis was supported when the measures assessed a person's degree of integration in a large social network. While such findings could be a function of methodology, both conceptualizations of social support appear to be correct. Each depicts a different process through which social support may enhance or attenuate health.

When applying the above social support hypotheses to childhood obesity, several issues are raised concerning the modification of the child's social milieu to effect weight change. Individual differences in need, desire, and availability of social support must be assessed (Cohen and Syme, 1985). The prudent clinician must ask:

A. Who is providing the support? The same resource may be acceptable from one provider but unacceptable from another. Positive comments regarding an adolescent female's change in body appearance may be quite acceptable from her family, but humiliating if received from male peers.

B. What kind of support is being provided? The specific resource must beneficially affect the child and be appropriate for the situation. For example, parental prompting of food selection may be appropriate for younger children and may be well received. However, in asserting their sense of self-mastery, teenagers may rebelliously eat whatever the parent did not prompt.

C. To whom is the support provided?   Is the child receptive to support? This can be influenced by the child's personality and social and cultural roles. The child must learn to attract and sustain support.

D. When is support provided?   Social support that may be effective at one point may be useless at another. Consider, for example, the child who has needed little praise, prompting or external guidance in the initial stages of weight loss. Two months after successful weight loss, the child begins to relapse. At this point, external support and problem solving may become crucial.

E. For how long is support provided?   While networks function well for short-term intervention, long-term support may stretch existing support structures beyond their capacity. If, for example, the obese child suffers from Prader-Willi syndrome, the tremendous support required by givers over a prolonged period is likely to create such a burden on the family that the support system disintegrates. Particularly for the chronically ill, the ability to sustain support or change existing patterns of support becomes a central issue.

F. What are the costs of giving and receiving support?   The perceived costs of asking for the receiving support may outweigh the perceived benefits of such support. A child from a lower socioeconomic single-parent household may not request more nutritious food items for fear of the increased expense it would create. She may not have her parent in attendance for treatment sessions because the already over-taxed parent cannot afford the time away from work and other family obligations.

Because social support is one predictor of successful treatment in obesity (Brownell, 1984), the clinician needs to contemplate how these support issues interact. If adequate support cannot be sustained throughout treatment or at crucial times in treatment, it may be best not to commence treatment until support needs are minimal or resources have increased.

IV.   Using the Social Arena to Aid the Obese Child in Weight Loss: Social Factors and Treatment

The etiology of adult obesity emerges from a combination of genetics and early childhood experiences with food and exercise, along with adult behavior (Brownell and Stunkard, 1980; Charney, Goodman, McBride,

Lyon and Pratt, 1976; Stunkard et al., 1986). Evidence suggests that impending obesity begins at ages six to nine years (Epstein, 1986; Shapiro et al., 1984). Such findings lead inevitably to the search for early interventions that will modify children's behavior and environment to reduce their risk for obesity and associated health risks. Environmental circumstances can be changed to increase frequency of supportive relationships in the endeavor to promote weight loss.

The social context in which a program is delivered may be as important as the nature of the program itself. Since eating and activity are often social events, attempts to maximize a child's support may be helpful, particularly for long-term success. Social factors involved in the treatment of obesity have been studied only recently. The results are encouraging. Most of the work with social support and childhood obesity has centered in two areas: Involving parents with their overweight children and school programs.

V. Family Interventions

If the social environment contributes to the genesis and/or maintenance of obesity, it is logical to treat obesity by altering the social environment. The family is the most obvious source of social influence. Parents exert a powerful influence on the eating, activity, and attitude patterns of their children. Parents model eating and physical activity patterns, control much of the food that enters the house, and establish an emotional environment in which thinness may or may not be encouraged. It is generally assumed that parents should be involved in the treatment of their obese children and that the parental role needs to be most structured for younger children. Since 1977 when Kingsley and Shapiro investigated the role of mothers in treatment, many studies have been conducted to determine what aspects of parental involvement are effective for particular age groups. When considered in light of developmental stages, parental involvement will vary in type and degree.

A. Treatment of Toddlers

One study has examined the effect of general health education with new mothers (Piscano, Lichter, Ritter and Siegal, 1978). Beginning when the children were 3 months old, an experimental group of mothers was instructed on the use of the "Prudent Diet", which was considerably lower in fat than the normal diet recommended in pediatric texts. The control group fed their children the normal diet. At age 3, significant differences were noted in the Prudent Diet group. The prevalence of obesity in the Prudent Diet group fell from 25% to 1%. The control group's prevalence rate remained elevated, beginning at 34% and ending at 26%.

Epstein, Wing and Valoski (in press) have just completed a one-year trial with 21 children ranging in age from one to five. The toddlers were given a family-based behavioral program to assess the feasibility of weight loss in youngsters with emphasis placed on nutrition and growth. In one year the average percentage of obesity decreased by 18.1%. No significant decrease in height percentile was found.

B. Obesity Programs for Five-year-olds through Teenagers

The majority of research assessing parental variables has been done with older children. The first controlled study in this area was reported by Kingsley and Shapiro (1977). Using 10- and 11-year-old children, the effects of involving or not involving mothers in treatment were examined. Weight losses did not differ in groups in which only the child attended, only the mother attended, or both the mother and child attended. However, satisfaction with the program was highest in the groups in which both mother and child attended.

An important distinction was made by Brownell, Kelman and Stunkard (1983) when they saw the parent and child together versus separately. These authors assessed whether parents would help or hinder their child's efforts to lose weight. There were 42 obese adolescents, ages 12–16, which were assigned randomly to one of three conditions: (a) Child Alone: Children attended groups alone, mothers were not involved; (b) Mother-Child Together: The children and mothers met together in the same group; and (c) Mother-Child Separately: The children and mothers both attended treatment sessions but met in separate groups. The mothers were not required to be overweight (73% were). The program included behavior modification, nutrition, exercise, cognitive restructuring, and special emphasis on family support.

After a 16-week program, the Mother-Child Separately group had lost more weight (18.5 lbs.) than the Mother-Child Together (11.7 lbs.) and the Child Alone (7.3 lbs.) groups. More dramatic results were noted at one-year follow-up. The latter two groups had regained to above their baseline weights, while the Mother-Child Separately group had essentially maintained their loss, as shown in Fig. 1.

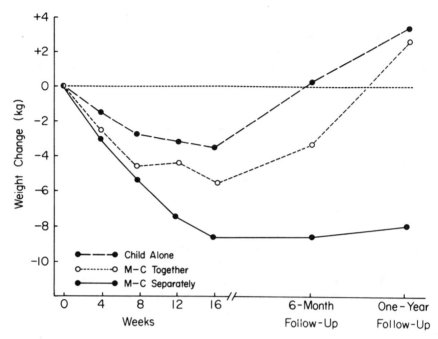

Fig. 1. Mean changes in weight for three treatment conditions (Child Alone, Mother-Child Together, Mother-Child Separately) during treatment and 1-year maintenance period. From Brownell, Kelman and Stunkard (1983).

When comparing the effects of treatment sessions with the parent and child together versus seeing the child alone, Coates, Killen and Slinkard (1982), like Brownell, Kelman and Stunkard (1983), found no significant differences at one-year follow-up.

Epstein et al. (1981 and in press) examined families in which both the parent and child were to lose weight versus the child alone versus a weight loss treatment with no specific target. All of the youngsters who reduced enough after eight months of behavior modification to fall beneath a mark of 20% overweight maintained this progress at one-year follow-up *if* their parents were treated also. In contrast, significantly fewer children (33%) given the same package but without their parents receiving the adult version of it were able to fall beneath the 20% overweight mark. In all of the groups, both the parent and the child were seen, but separately. At five-year follow-up, children in the parent-plus-child group maintained their weight loss, whereas, children in the other groups approached baseline or above. Of the children in the parent and child group 42% were no longer obese, while only 19% and 4% of the children in the other two groups were not obese. This long-term effect strongly suggests the desirability of including the parent as an active member in the treatment of childhood obesity.

In contrast, Israel, Stolmaker, Sharp, Silverman and Simon (1984) examined the issue of whether parallel parental weight loss was a necessary component of involvement. They provided the parents of the overweight children with a choice of either engaging in a weight loss program like their children's or improving their skills as a helper. Both types of parental involvement were equally successful in producing weight loss for their children during treatment and at one-year follow-up.

Next, Israel, Stolmaker and Andrian (1985) addressed the importance of parental behavior change in the process of treating obese children. Two conditions were compared. Families were assigned either to a weight reduction only condition, receiving a multicomponent behavioral weight control program, or to a parent training group which received the same treatment plus a course on child management skills. Maintenance of weight loss was superior for the children in the parent training condition at one-year follow-up. Since the study did not evaluate behavioral changes in child management practices, it remains to be determined what specific changes in parental behavior accounted for the greater degree of success.

Coates and Thoresen (1981) have used single-subject design to investigate the effects of behavior modification on weight control for three teenagers. One subject served as a control and did not receive treatment. The program included self-monitoring, stimulus control, modification of eating behavior, exercise management, and reinforcement. The experimenters worked with the families and carefully analyzed the eating and food-storage habits in the home. An association between specific behavior changes and weight change was demonstrated. The experimental subjects lost 21 and 11.5 pounds. The control subject gained five pounds.

Kirschenbaum, Harris and Tomarken (1984) examined the effect of parental involvement on aspects other than weight. Children in a child-plus-parent group (both the child and parent attended sessions) and the child only group (where parents were given homework but did not attend treatment sessions) lost significant amounts of weight and maintained these losses at one-year follow-up. However, the parent plus child group showed no attrition versus a 50% drop out rate in the child alone group. Weight loss of parents in the parent-child group was greater than for the child alone group.

The above findings are encouraging. These losses rank among the highest in the treatment of childhood obesity. Of particular note is the success of the children in the Mother-Child Separately group in maintenance of weight loss (Brownell et al. 1983, Epstein et al., in press).

These studies illustrate that a subtle change in the approach used with the parents (having the mother meet together with or separately from her child and/or have the parent involved in his/her own adult weight loss or child management program conjointly with the child) had a powerful effect on weight loss. As shown in the other studies, having the mothers involved offered no advantage to having the children meet alone, except when the mother and children were involved in separate meetings.

These studies have only touched on parental and family factors in the treatment of childhood obesity. Because the role of parental involvement is crucial in the child's energy intake and expenditure, this issue will remain open to systematic research in order to enhance and prolong treatment effects. Differences in the degree and type of parental partici- pation among these studies indicate that it is premature to draw firm conclusions. More research is needed to define clearly the nature of the parent's role and the specific skills which the parents need to aid their overweight children.

VI. Treatment in the Schools

We cover treatment in the schools briefly to emphasize the perspective of the broad social system and powerful social resources in the school. The reader should refer to Guy Parcel's chapter on school programs in this volume for in-depth coverage of this topic.

The interventions presented in the previous section were designed for clinical use, and, consequently, they are applied to only a small number of obese children. There are several important advantages to treating obesity in the schools. First, large numbers of children can be screened, treated, monitored, and followed longitudinally. Second, cost to the family can be minimized. Third, the child becomes a participant in an educational experience rather than acquiring the status of patient from the medical arena. Finally, from a preventive perspective, children who are not obese or only mildly overweight, or not overweight at all but are at risk because of obese parents, can be identified and instructed in appropriate eating and exercise habits before problems become serious enough to warrant professional attention.

Given the promise in this area, increasing numbers of studies are being reported. The most thoroughly evaluated school programs have been set forth by Seltzer and Mayer (1970), Botvin, Cantlon, Carter and Williams (1979), Collipp (1980), Lansky and Brownell (1982), Lansky and Vance (1983), Foster, Wadden and Brownell (1985), and Brownell and Kaye

(1982). All reported significant weight losses in programs combining behavior modification, exercise, nutrition, and social support. However, with the exception of Brownell and Kaye (1982), the weight losses were small, and long-term evaluation was not conducted.

Brownell and Kaye (1982) carried out a school program for obese children five through twelve years old which involved instruction in nutrition, behavior modification, exercise, and social support. Figure 2 depicts the model which guided the program. Behavioral techniques were emphasized as a means for encouraging changes in nutrition and activity levels. Equally important was the context in which the program was administered to best foster social support. The program was designed to enhance support to the child from a number of important sources, including parents, teachers, and peers.

Ninety-five percent of the children lost weight, despite the weight gain that was expected due to maturation. Treatment children demonstrated an average decrease in percent overweight of 15.4% while the control group became heavier. The magnitude of the changes was on a par with

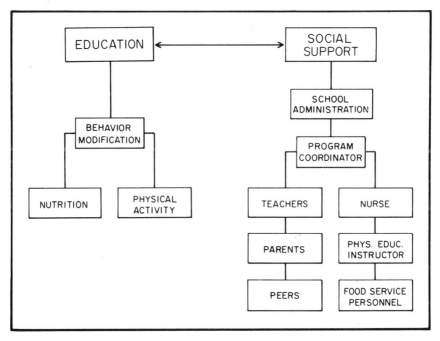

Fig. 2. The conceptual model for a program of weight control in the schools. The model emphasizes the process by which the program is implemented (social support), as well as the program components (education). From Brownell and Kaye (1982).

weight losses observed in clinical settings. The authors reported anecdotally that social support factors seemed central to the program's success. The program coordinator (a nurse's aide) conducted the program in such a positive light that thin children wanted to participate. All of the participating children's names were prominently posted, and an awards ceremony was held before the entire school in which the children were given certificates. Anticipated stigma against the overweight children did not occur.

Foster et al. (1985) expanded the school program to include older peer counselors. While the weight losses in this program were statistically significant, clinical significance was marginal (mean loss at 18-week follow-up of 0.67 lbs.). In terms of social impact, however, it was found that the self-concept in the program children improved significantly. Factors other than weight loss can be assessed when evaluating weight-loss programs.

To summarize, the initial findings in school programs are promising, but before we can embrace this approach, more research needs to be done. Experimental control has not been evidenced in most cases, weight losses have been small, and only short-term results are available. In light of the potential benefits of school intervention, this area is a direction in which the field could focus its efforts in order to reach the greatest number of children.

VII. Conclusions

Childhood obesity is a serious public health problem. It predisposes a child to serious medical disorders in adult life. For many obese persons, the psychological and social consequences of being fat are worse than the medical implications.

We have outlined the function of social support both in its contribution to the development of obesity and to its management. The role of social support has shown promising results for children in school settings and in the clinic. Although neither area has received enough examination to draw firm conclusions, it does appear that changes in both arenas can facilitate behavior changes in intake and activity patterns.

From a biobehavioral perspective, social, genetic, and physiological factors are central to the etiology of obesity. It appears that if earlier identification of high risk children occurs (i.e., those who are already obese or have obese parents) and/or preventive measures can be taken (Piscano et al., 1978), the incidence of obesity could be curtailed. Epstein's work suggests that significant changes can be effected in the first five years of life (see his chapter in this volume). The other studies showed significant clinical improvement in middle and late childhood obesity.

The implications of the research surveyed throughout this chapter suggest that there is potential for powerful intervention in important settings. There is reason to be optimistic, but not complacent. Many issues must be addressed before public health implications of these programs are clear. Among these issues are the degree to which parents, older peer counselors, and schools can and should be involved, the nature of maintenance strategies which might be implemented, and the extent to which psychological and social factors change as a result of participation in such programs. Furthermore, the interrelationship between social, physiological and genetic factors needs to be examined. For example, how do socio-economic and ethnic variables interrelate with family-feeding practices and what effect do these relationships have on number and size of fat cells in early, middle and late childhood? One can imagine the day when well-baby clinics are the primary settings for reducing the incidence of obesity.

References

Allon, N. (1979). Self-perceptions of the stigma of overweight in relationship to weight-losing patterns. *American Journal of Clinical Nutrition*, *32*, 470–480.

Birch, L. (1979a). Preschool children's food preferences and consumption patterns. *Journal of Nutrition Education*, *11*, 189–192.

Birch, L. (1979b). Dimensions of preschool children's food preferences. *Journal of Nutrition Education*, *11*, 77–80.

Birch, L. (1980). Effects of peer models' food choices and eating behaviors on pre-schoolers' food preferences. *Child Development*, *51*, 489–496.

Birch, L. & Marlin, D. (1982). I don't like it; I never tried it: Effects of exposure on two-year-old children's food preferences. *Appetite: Journal of Intake Research*, *3*, 353–360.

Birch, L., Zimmerman, S. & Hind, H. (1980). The influence of social affective context on the formation of children's food preferences. *Child Development*, *51*, 856–861.

Botvin, G., Cantlon, A., Carter, B. & Williams, C. (1979). Reducing adolescent obesity through a school health program. *Journal of Pediatrics*, *95*, 1060–1062.

Broadhead, W., Kaplan, B., James, S., Wagner, E., Schoenbach, V., Grimsom, R., Heyden, S., Tibblin, G. & Gehlbach, S. (1983). The epidemiologic evidence for a relationship between social support and health. *American Journal of Epidemiology*, *117*, 521–537.

Brownell, K. (1982). Obesity: Understanding and treating a serious, prevalent and refractory disorder. *Journal of Consulting and Clinical Psychology*, *50*, 820–840.

Brownell, K. (1984). Behavioral, psychological and environmental predictors of obesity and success at weight reduction. *International Journal of Obesity*, *8*, 543–550.

Brownell, K. (1984). The psychology and physiology of obesity: Implications for screening and treatment. *Journal of the American Dietetic Association*, *84*(4), 406–414.

Brownell, K. (1986). Social and behavioral aspects of obesity in children, In Krasnegor, N., Arasteh, J. & Cataldo, M., (Eds.) *Child Health Behavior: A Behavioral Pediatrics Perspective*, N.Y., John Wiley & Sons.

Brownell, K. & Kaye, F. (1982). A school based behavior modification, nutrition education, and physical activity program for obese children. *American Journal of Clinical Nutrition*, 35, 277–283.

Brownell, K., Kelman, J. & Stunkard, A. (1983). Treatment of obese children with and without their mothers: Changes in weight and blood pressure. *Pediatrics*, 71, 515–523.

Brownell, K. & Stunkard, A. (1978). Behavioral treatment of obesity in children. *American Journal of Disabled Children*, 132, 403.

Brownell, K. & Stunkard, A. (1980). Physical activity in the development and control of obesity. In Stunkard, A. (Ed.), *Obesity*. Philadelphia: Saunders.

Canning, H. & Mayer, J. (1966). Obesity: Its possible effects on college acceptance. *New England Journal of Medicine*, 275, 1172–1174.

Charney, E., Goodman, H., Mc Bride, M., Lyon, B. & Pratt, R., (1976). Childhood antecedents of adult obesity: Do chubby infants become obese adults? *New England Journal of Medicine, 295*, 6–9.

Coates, T., Killen, J. & Slinkard, L. (1982). Parent participation in a treatment program for overweight adolescents. *International Journal of Eating Disorders*, 1, 37–48.

Coates, T. & Thoresen, C. (1981). Behavior and weight changes in three obese adolescents. *Behavior Research Therapy*, 12, 383–399.

Cohen, S. & Syme, L. (1985). *Social Support and Health*. Orlando, Florida: Academic Press, Inc.

Cohen, S. & Wills, T. (1985). Stress, social support and the buffering hypothesis. *Psychological Bulletin*, 98, 310–357.

Collipp, P. (1980). Obesity programs in public schools. In *Childhood Obesity*, 2nd Edition, edited by P. Collipp, pp. 297–308. Massachusetts: PSG Publishing Company.

Dietz, W. & Gortmaker, S. (1985). Do we fatten our children at the television set: Obesity and television viewing in children and adolescents. *Pediatrics*, 75, 807–812.

Edelman, B. (1982). Developmental differences in the conceptualization of obesity: A preliminary analysis of elementary school children's responses. *Journal of American Dietetics Association*, 80, page 122.

Epstein, L. (1986). Treatment of childhood obesity. In *Handbook of Eating Disorders*, Brownell, K. & Foreyt, J. (Eds.). NY: Basic Books, Inc.

Epstein, L., Masek, B. & Marshall, W. (1978). A nutritionally based school program for control of eating in obese children. *Behavior Therapy*, 9, 766–788.

Epstein, L., Wing, R., Koeske, R., Andrasik, F. & Ossip, D. (1981). Child and parent weight loss in family based behavior modification programs. *Journal of Consulting and Clinical Psychology*, 49, 674–685.

Epstein, L., Wing, R. & Valoski, A. (1987). Long-term effects of family-based treatment of childhood obesity. *Journal of Consulting and Clinical Psychology*, 55, 91–95.

Epstein, L., Woodall, K., Goreczny, A., Wing, R. & Robertson, R. (1984). The modification of activity patterns and energy expenditure in obese young girls. *Behavior Therapy*, 15, 101–108.

Foman, S. (1974). *Infant Nutrition*. Philadelphia: W.B. Saunders.

Foster, G., Wadden, T. & Brownell, K. (1985). Peer-led program for the treatment and prevention of obesity in the schools. *Journal of Consulting and Clinical Psychology*, 53, 538–540.

Harper, L. & Sanders, K. (1975). The effect of adults eating on young children's acceptance of unfamiliar food. *Journal of Experimental Child Psychology*, 20, 206–214.

Herbert-Jackson, E., Cross, M. & Risley, T. (1977). Milk types and temperature: What will young children drink? *Journal of Nutrition Education*, 9, 76–79.

Israel, A. C. & Shapiro, L. S. (1985). Behavior problems of obese children enrolling in a weight-reduction program. *Journal of Pediatric Psychology*, 10, 449–460.

Israel, A. C., Stolmaker, L. & Andrian, C. (1985). The effects of training parents in general child management skills on a behavioral weight loss program for children. *Behavior Therapy*, *16*, 169−180.

Israel, A. C., Stolmaker, L., Sharp, J., Silverman, W. & Simon, L. (1984). An evaluation of two methods of parental involvement in treating obese children. *Behavior Therapy*, *15*, 266−272.

Kingsley, R. & Shapiro, J. (1977). A comparison of three behavioral programs for control of obesity. *Behavior Therapy*, *8*, 30−36.

Kirschenbaum, D., Harris, E. & Tomarken, A. (1984). Effects of parental involvement in behavioral weight loss therapy for preadolescents. *Behavior Therapy*, *15*, 485−500.

Klesges, R. (1984). Personality and obesity: Global versus specific measures? *Behavioral Assessment*, *6*, 347−356.

Klesges, R., Malott, J., Boschee, P. & Weber, J. (1986). The effects of parental influences on children's food intake, physical activity and relative weight. *International Journal of Eating Disorders*, *5*, 335−345.

Klesges, R., Coates, T., Brown, G., Sturgeon-Tillisch, Moldenhauer-Klesges, L., Holzer, B., Woolfrey, J. & Vollmer, J. (1983). Parental influences on children's eating behavior and relative weight. *Journal of Applied Behavior Analysis*, *16*, 371−378.

Klesges, R., Coates, T., Moldenhauer-Klesges, L., Holzer, B., Gustavson, J. & Barnes, J. (1984). An observational system for assessing physical activity in children and associated parent behavior. *Behavioral Assessment*, *6*, 333−345.

Kolata, G. (1986). Obese children: A growing problem. *Science*, *232*, 20−21.

Lansky, D. & Brownell, K. (1982). Comparison of school-based treatments for adolescent obesity. *Journal of School Health*, *8*, 384−387.

Lansky, D. & Vance, M. (1983). School-based intervention for adolescent obesity: Analysis of treatment, randomly selected control, and self-selected subjects. *Journal of Consulting and Clinical Psychology*, *51*, 147−148.

Leavy, R. (1983). Social support and psychological disorder: A review. *Journal of Community Psychology*, *11*, 3−21.

Maddox, G., Back, K. & Liederman, V. (1968). Overweight as social deviance and disability. *Journal of Health and Social Behavior*, *9*, 287.

Marinho, H. (1942). Social influence in the formation of enduring preferences. *Journal of Abnormal and Social Psychology*, *37*, 448−468.

McCarthy, D. (1935). Children's feeding problems in relation to the food aversions of the family. *Child Development*, *6*, 277−284.

Mendelson, B. & White, D. (1982). Relation between body-esteem and self-esteem of obese and normal children. *Perceptual and Motor Skills*, *54*, 899−905.

Mendelson, B. & White, D. (1985). Development of Self-Body-Esteem in overweight youngsters. *Developmental Psychology*, *21*, 90−96.

Mitchell, R., Billings, A. & Moos, R. (1982). Social support and well-being: Implications for prevention programs. *Journal of Primary Prevention*, *3*, 77−98.

Monello, L. & Mayer, J. (1963). Obese adolescent girls: An unrecognized minority group? *American Journal of Clinical Nutrition*, *13*, 35−39.

Perry, R., LeBow, M. & Buser, M. (1979). An exploration of observational learning in modifying selected eating responses in obese children. *International Journal of Obesity*, *3*, 193−199.

Piscano, J., Lichter, H., Ritter, J. & Siegal, A. (1978). An attempt at prevention of obesity in infancy. *Pediatrics*, *61*, 360−364.

Sallade, J. (1973). A comparison of psychological adjustment of obese versus non-obese children. *Journal of Psychosomatic Research*, *17*, 89−96.

Sarason, I., Levine, H., Basham, R. & Sarason, B. (1983). Assessing social support: The social support questionnaire. *Journal of Personality and Social Psychology, 44,* 127–139.

Seltzer, C. & Mayer, J. (1970). An effective weight control program in a public school system. *American Journal of Public Health, 60,* 679–689.

Shapiro, L., Crawford, P., Clark, M., Pearson, D., Raz, J. & Huenemann, R. (1984). Obesity prognosis: A longitudinal study of children from the age of 6 months to 9 years. *American Journal of Public Health, 74,* 968–972.

Staffieri, J. (1967). A study of social stereotype of body image in children. *Journal of Personality and Social Psychology, 7,* 101–104.

Stark, L. J., Collins, F. L., Jr., Osnes, P. G., Stokes, T. F. (1986). Using reinforcement and cueing to increase healthy snack food choices in preschoolers. *Journal of Applied Behavior Analysis 19,* 367–379.

Stunkard, A. (1975). From explanation to action in psychosomatic medicine: The case of obesity. *Psychosomatic Medicine, 37,* 195–236.

Stunkard, A. (1976). *The Pain of Obesity,* Palo Alto, CA: Bull Publishing Co.

Stunkard, A., Sorensen, T., Hanis, C., Teasdale, M., Chakraborty, R., Schull, W. & Schulsinger, F. (1986). An adoption study of human obesity. *New England Journal of Medicine, 314,* 193–198.

Wadden, T., Foster, G., Brownell, K. & Finley, E. (1984). Self-concept in obese and normal-weight children, *Journal of Consulting and Clinical Psychology, 52,* 1104–1105.

Wadden, T. & Stunkard, A. (1985). Social and psychological consequences of obesity. *Annals of Internal Medicine, 103,* 1062–1067.

Waxman, M. & Stunkard, A. (1980). Caloric intake and expenditure of obese boys. *Journal of Pediatrics, 96,* 187–193.

II

DETERMINANTS

3

Genetic and Familial Factors in Human Obesity[1]

R.M. SIERVOGEL
Division of Human Biology, Department of Pediatrics,
School of Medicine,
Wright State University
Yellow Springs, Ohio

I. Introduction

The definite and conspicuous familial aggregation that occurs with obesity has been recognized since well before the turn of the century (Rony, 1940). It was, no doubt, this observation that first interested geneticists in obesity as a genetic trait. While there is strong evidence for the familial nature of obesity, surprisingly little is known about specific genetic mechanisms involved. Even the early geneticists realized that the familial nature of the problem did not necessarily result from genetic causes. There is a large literature relating to heredity and obesity, but only recently has the relative importance of genetic and environmental factors in this trait been addressed in a very rigorous manner.

This paper summarizes some of the research that has been done in the area of familial and genetic factors affecting obesity, and, as such, it reviews approaches that have been used in the past for studying this question. Some of the problems associated with investigating this trait are discussed, and suggestions are made for approaches that could be used in future research into the genetics of obesity. The paper does not deal with the important and relevant area relating to the use of animal models in investigating this subject. These have been reviewed elsewhere (Bray and York, 1971; Greenwood et al., 1979; Bray, 1984; Trayhurn, 1984).

[1] This work was supported in part by a research grant from the National Institute of Child Health and Human Development (HDAM-R01-12252).

Several reviews, at least in part, cover the genetic contribution to obesity in humans (Rony, 1940; Bruch, 1957; Seltzer, 1967; Mayer, 1960, 1968; Mann, 1974; Greenwood, et al., 1979; Mueller, 1983; Bray, 1984). In order to present a balanced perspective, consideration is given to some of the more classical studies of genetic and familial factors in obesity before focusing attention on more modern approaches to studying this problem.

II Classical Studies of the Genetics of Obesity

A. Family Studies

1. *An early comprehensive study* Davenport (1923) carried out one of the first and more detailed of the early genetic studies. He studied numerous multigenerational families involving over 500 matings. Individuals were classified into five categories from "very slender" to "very fleshy" on the basis of an index (Weight/Stature^2, W/S^2). This categorization is an example of one problem encountered with virtually all genetic studies to date. Because of the lack of appropriate analytic methodology to deal with quantitative traits, investigators divided continuous variables into dichotomies (at worst) or into several categories (at best). Another problem with Davenport's study is that he did not correct for age, although he did limit his study to individuals over 18 years of age. He noted, however: "In adult life the changes in build vary with families. In those characterized by slender build there is typically little change. In those characterized by fleshy build there is typically progressive increase in weight to 50 years."

Davenport (1923) found that slender x slender matings produced relatively few nonslender progeny, whereas matings between two fleshy individuals produced a much higher proportion of nonfleshy offspring. That is, there was an almost doubled amount of variability among progeny from obese matings compared to those from slender matings. In three generation pedigrees, he found that the progeny who came from obese × slender matings were more variable than progeny of obese parents from obese × obese matings or slender parents from slender × slender matings. From these and similar findings, Davenport concluded that Mendelian segregation occurred in these families. He proposed that at least three independent genes were involved and that the alleles for obesity tended to be dominant to the nonobese alleles. Thus, slender individuals tend to be homozygous, whereas obese persons are often heterozygous. This hypothesis was the first and probably the most specific that has been suggested for the hereditary component of "obesity" in humans. However, it was not unequivocally substantiated by his data, nor those from any later study.

2. *Familial nature of obesity* One observation that has been made repeatedly is that fat people generally have at least one fat parent. Bouchard (1882) and van Noorden (1907), cited in Rony (1940) found that 50 to 60% of patients with "constitutional" obesity have obese parents. Dunlop et al. (1931) observed in their sample of over 500 individuals from 15 to 141% overweight, that 39% had only a fat mother, 12% had only a fat father and 18% had both parents fat. Ellis and Tallerman (1934), in a sample of 50 obese children aged 5 to 14 years, found 26% had an obese mother, 12% had an obese father and 6% had both parents obese. In another 16 percent there were obese siblings, but parents of normal weight. Gurney (1936) found that of 61 "stout" women, 43% had a stout mother, 15% had a stout father and 25% had both parents stout. In a control group of 47 nonstout women, 30% had a stout mother, 2% had a stout father and 6% had both parents stout. In Rony's (1940) study of 250 obese individuals, 69% had at least one obese parent while 24% had two obese parents. In a sample of 116 white females, Angel (1949) found that 36% had fat mothers, 16% had fat fathers and 26% had both parents fat. Numerous other investigators have made similar observations (Fellows, 1931; Bauer, 1945; Iversen, 1953; Johnson, 1956; Mayer, 1960; Withers, 1964). Both Gurney (1936) and Angel (1949) considered Mendelian segregation was occurring in their study families, but they did not speculate as to the number of genes and the dominance relationships of these genes.

That obesity has a familial nature is indicated also by the findings of Mossberg (1948), who was interested particularly in the age of onset of obesity. In his sample of 493 obese individuals, Mossberg observed that those from families with more than one obese person became obese before 6 years more commonly than did those from families with only one obese member. Mullins (1958) found obesity was more common in the near relatives of individuals who became obese as a juvenile than in relatives of individuals who became obese as adults. Whether these patterns are due to genetic or environmental causes is unclear.

Vamberova et al. (1968), in a study of 334 families ascertained through obese probands and 563 families ascertained through normal probands, computed risk figures for obesity. They concluded that the probability of obesity in a sibling of a proband was 0.2 if the mother was obese and 0.25 if both parents were obese. In addition, they found that 14% of the obese individuals had two nonobese parents, 49% had one obese parent and 47% had two obese parents. These figures taken from a Czechoslovakian population agree almost exactly with those of Withers (1964) derived from a British population.

Romaniuk-Michalska and Krotkiewski (1969) did a rather detailed study of the families of 375 obese individuals (mostly women). The family incidence of obesity in this sample was similar to that in previous studies. They concluded that their data supported a hypothesis of an important hereditary component in the etiology of obesity, but that no simple Mendelian pattern existed. They stated there was a need for studies "that cover ... not only obese patients, but also persons of normal weight chosen from several successive generations." They made two noteworthy observations: (1) successive generations displayed a predisposition to identical topography of fatty tissue; and (2) obesity appears earlier and is more marked in individuals with a family history of obesity. That they recognized the need to study the genetics of the topography of fatty tissue, i.e., fat patterning, is significant because this is an area of current interest.

3. *Familial correlations* Heritability, loosely defined, is the proportion of the variation in a trait due to genetic causes. In samples ascertained through fat women and women unselected for fat, Withers (1961) estimated the heritability of "log percentage overweight" as 0.29 using mother-offspring regression in the control population. He calculated the sib-sib intraclass correlation to be 0.26. Heritability using the father-offspring regression was estimated to be 0.55. The wide variability of the heritability indices exemplify the problems associated with interpreting these indices in human beings. Another factor that must be considered when interpreting Withers' data is that the weights of relatives were obtained from questionnaires.

Reynolds (1951), using a sample of children enrolled in The Fels Longitudinal Growth Study aged 6.5 or 7.5 years, briefly discussed hereditary factors in certain measurements of subcutaneous fat. The sample sizes he used to calculate various statistics were small, generally in the 15 to 50 range. In measurements of fat breadth in calf, waist and forearm, he found that closely related pairs tend to be more similar to each other than more distantly related or unrelated pairs. In computing parent-child, parent-parent and brother-sister correlations for fat breadth in chest and calf, he used the 6.5- and 7.5-year-old children and their parents at whatever age they had been examined. The only significant correlations were 0.39 and 0.48 between father and son for calf and chest fat breadth respectively. There is questionable biological significance to these findings, primarily because of small sample sizes and large age discrepancies for which no corrections were made.

Garn et al. (1975), using measurements of lateral thoracic fatfold from a sample of the Pre-School Nutrition Survey of the U.S.A., found high positive sibling correlations (about 0.3). It is not clear, however, whether they are due to genetic or environmental causes. Using a sample from the Ten State Nutrition Survey of the U.S.A., they have shown that, for subscapular and triceps fatfolds, there are high parent-child correlations (about 0.3); however, they found a marital correlation of about the same magnitude. Using data from the Tecumseh (Michigan) project of the University of Michigan School of Public Health, they again found that the marital correlation was similar to the sibling correlations (about 0.25), indicating that "genetically-unrelated subjects are about as similar, fatwise, as genetically-related individuals." Thus it appears that people living together have a similarity in degree of fatness. The authors point out, however, that these data "do not reject the genetic hypothesis, but they do indicate the need for more sophisticated (research) designs."

The finding of an aggregation of obesity in families where there is a biological relationship but an absence of aggregation in adoptive families is highly suggestive of a prominent genetic involvement in the manifestation of this trait. Also, the finding that positive correlations are found consistently for fat measures in related individuals supports this hypothesis. However, like Garn et al. (1975), not all studies are strongly supportive of genetic involvement. For example, Matsuki and Yoda (1971) found that while the parents of 374 Japanese college women showed a significant correlation (mother versus father) for weight, none existed for height. This suggests an environmental effect or assortative mating. Matsuki and Yoda (1971) examined parent-daughter correlations for only one college age daughter in each family and their analysis was performed on weight expressed as a percent deviation from a standard previously developed for Japanese (Matsuki et al., 1971). They concluded that, while height is influenced strongly by genetic predisposition, weight is mostly influenced by environment.

4. *Social inheritance* To determine if "social inheritance" was confounded with genetic inheritance and manifesting itself as dominance, Withers (1964) studied adoptive families and families ascertained through school children about the same age as the adopted children. For "percentage overweight" he did not find a significant correlation between adoptees and their adoptive parents, indicating that genetic, not environmental, causes accounted for the similarities between relatives. In natural children, he found significant father-daughter, mother-daughter and mother-son correlations. Initially, he considered that the pattern was suggestive of sex-limited inheritance, but more detailed analyses of his

data lead him to abandon the hypothesis. Withers concluded, after this extensive familial correlation study, that percentage overweight is unsatisfactory as a phenotype in the study of the genetics of obesity.

5. *Studies in a population isolate* In a study of a Hutterite religious isolate, Martin et al. (1973) made a genetic survey of various anthropological variables including several relevant to obesity. There is extensive inbreeding among the individuals in this population and they share a relatively uniform environment, because of their communal life-style established by religious dictates. Multiple regression of each variable with age, degree of completeness of the pedigree (extensive pedigree records go back to 1700), and the inbreeding coefficient were performed. Although there were many small but significant relationships between certain variables and the inbreeding coefficient, their biological importance is unclear. Residuals were used in familial correlation studies. Marital, parental and sibling correlations were calculated; cholesterol, weight, height, skinfold thickness and diastolic blood pressure showed a pattern of marital correlation zero and parental and sibling correlations that were significantly different from zero (all positive). This is the pattern expected on genetic grounds and would be difficult to explain, in this population, on the basis of environmental causes. Inbreeding, which tends to increase homozygosity, was found to have an effect on the anthropological measurements (decreasing skeletal measurements; increasing measurements of fat). Martin et al. (1973) state that "this might indicate that homozygosity ... reduces the ability of the body to handle fat deposition." In addition they point out, "that there is genetic control over obesity in this population is also suggested by the pattern of familial correlations for weight and skinfold thickness."

B. Twin Studies

It has been shown that, of a multitude of anthropological measurements made on identical twins, weight generally is the most variable (Von Verschuer, 1927; Newman et al., 1937). As might be expected, monozygotic twins raised in different environments show about three times more variation in weight than those raised in the same environment. Although weight is one of the measurements most sensitive to environmental influences, it still appears to show a large genetic influence. Newman et al. (1937) reported that dizygotic twins have the same variability with respect to weight as do same-sex non-twin sibs, and that both these groups are about 2½ times more variable than monozygotic twins. In addition, 19 pairs of monozygotic twins separated in early childhood average age at observation 26 years) generally showed small

differences in weight. The correlation for weight was very high in monozygotic twins raised together (0.97). Others have also found closer similarities in body fatness between monozygotic than between dizygotic
twins (Feinleib et al., 1977).

Gordon (1957), in a comparison between monozygotic twins reared
separately and others reared together, found those reared together varied
by only 3%, indicating a significant genetic influence. Tanner (1955), in a
similar study, demonstrated that for weight and certain other measurements,
the intraclass correlation coefficients for monozygotic twins reared together
and those for monozygotic twins reared apart are virtually identical. Both
coefficients are much higher than those for sibs and nonidentical twins.
"In other words, body weight is fundamentally and to a very great degree
controlled by genetic factors" (Tanner, 1955).

Clark (1956), using about 40 pairs of adolescent mono- and dizygotic
twins, calculated a heritability estimate of 0.69 for body weight. Similar
estimates have been obtained by others: 0.78 (Newman et al., 1937), 0.83
(Burt, 1966). Osborne and De George (1959) did not find a high heritability
for body weight in their sample of 50 to 60 pairs of adult mono- and
dizygotic twins. However, they did find that subscapular skinfold thickness
seemed to have a significant genetic component. In addition, they concluded
that somatotype ratings reflected genetic control, including a strong factor
of sex influence. This also was observed by Withers (1964).

C. Other Studies in Humans

Seltzer and Mayer (1964) reported that obese adolescent girls differ
from their nonobese counterparts in tending to be more endomorphic,
more mesomorphic and less ectomorphic. Seltzer (1967) states "from the
anthropological data, it would appear that there are constitutional and
genetic factors operating in the predisposition to obesity."

Steatopygia of Bushman and Hottentot women is a form of localized
adipose tissue accumulation that is directly under genetic control (Mayer,
1968). There are genetic diseases in which a component of the syndrome
is an accumulation of abnormal fats or normal fat in localized parts of the
body or, in some cases, all over the body. These include Niemann-Pick
syndrome, Tay Sachs disease, Hand-Schuller-Christian syndrome and
Gaucher's disease (Mayer, 1968). Single genes can, and do, result in
obesity either directly or indirectly.

In addition to obesity occurring as part of a genetic syndrome, Mayer
(1968) cites several other, probably genetic, diseases in which a major
finding is obesity. In macrosomia adiposa congenita, which is usually
lethal by age 1 year, the affected individuals develop gross obesity soon

after birth, accompanied by marked voracity and precocious skeletal development. McKusick (1975) has catalogued this condition as autosomal recessive. In familial monstrous infantile obesity, overeating does not become striking until several months of age.

D. Summary

The genetic studies that followed Davenport's pioneering efforts have been characterized by Steinberg (1960) as "anecdotal, i.e., isolated pedigrees not critically examined." Although this perhaps seems like a rather harsh criticism and an overgeneralization, there is appreciable truth to it, especially in regard to specific genetic mechanisms. Steinberg's characterization applies also to many of the studies made during the past 26 years. However, we should point out that, unlike Davenport's work, the genetic/familial aspect of most published studies of obesity has been an aside, rather than the central theme of the research study.

There are definite genetic factors related to obesity in man; however, this does not necessarily imply that "ordinary" obesity is under strict genetic control. The most convincing evidence for specific genetic causes of obesity come from animal studies in which major gene and polygenic cases are known to exist (Bray and York, 1971; Greenwood et al., 1979; Bray, 1984; Trayhurn, 1984). Two points are clear: 1) Genetic factors play an important role in many aspects of body build. The effects of these factors can be seen in gross measurements (such as weight) as well as measurements (e.g., cholesterol levels) closer to the biochemical pathways that must be involved. 2) Few, if any, really adequate genetic studies have been done to date. This is partially because only recently has the methodology for dealing properly with certain aspects of quantitative traits become available.

III. Recent Studies of the Genetics of Obesity

Genetic and environmental factors can be dissected from one another using data from families with adopted individuals. Data from the Danish Adoption Register (Schulsinger, et al., 1985) has been used for this purpose. Stunkard et al. (1986) used self-reported weight and stature data from 540 adoptees and their biological and adoptive parents selected from the 3580 who originally responded to a mailed questionnaire. These adoptees were selected to be in one of four weight categories representing the range of weight from thin to obese. W/S^2, an index of obesity, was used as the variable of interest. The results indicated that across all weight classes there was no relation between the weight class of the adoptees and W/S^2 of their adoptive parents, but there was a strong relationship between the weight class of the adoptees and W/S^2 of biological parents. Stunkard et al. (1986) concluded that genetic influences have a much greater role than family environment in determining fatness.

W/S^2 constructed from self-reported weight and stature tends to be an underestimation of true W/S^2, because of a systematic overestimation of stature and underestimation of weight, even though individually self-reported estimates of weight and stature have a high degree of accuracy (Stewart et al., 1987). However this phenomenon would have little effect on the conclusions of Stunkard et al. (1986).

Path analysis has also been used to separate environmental and genetic influences in obesity-related traits. For data from Muscatine, Iowa, Hanis et al. (1983) used path models in which genetic, common household and individual environmental effects were among the parameters of the model. They found a heritability of 0.15 for weight, which is lower than estimates of some other studies. For example, Rao et al. (1975) reported heritability of 0.44 for weight in pedigrees from northeastern Brazil and Bouchard et al. (1980) reported values near 0.3 for a sample of Canadians.

In an investigation of W/S^2 and stature in the Framingham Heart Study, Heller, et al. (1984) used serial data collected from individuals in about 1949 and again in the early 1970s. They found that the pattern of familial correlations showed a marked familial resemblance for W/S^2 among first degree relatives, but did not favor a large genetic contribution to this similarity. These conclusions are similar in part to those of Hawk and Brook (1979), Karlin et al. (1981), Rona (1981), and Khoury et al. (1983). On the other hand, most studies seem to support strongly a pronounced genetic component in obesity-related traits (e.g., Savard, et al., 1983; Bouchard et al., 1985).

IV. A Genetic-Epidemiological Approach to Investigating Obesity

Modern methods of genetic epidemiology provide means for better determining and separating genetic and environmental factors affecting traits such as obesity. These approaches have been reviewed (Curnow and Smith, 1975; Elston and Rao, 1978; Boyle and Elston, 1979; Cloninger et al., 1983), and books covering the recent methodological developments are now available. These emphasize different aspects of genetic epidemiology, including general aspects (Morton, 1982; Morton et al. 1983), genetic linkage analysis (Ott, 1984), and genealogical inference (Thompson, 1985).

Recent studies have tended to focus on developing extensions to variance component models (Lange et al., 1976), path analysis (Cloninger et al., 1983) and to a greater extent the likelihood model described by Elston and Stewart (1971). In addition, practical and comprehensive regressive models have been proposed by Bonney (1984, 1986). These models can be used to summarize family data with or without specifying a particular genetic mechanism of transmission.

There are a variety of approaches to analyzing genetic mechanisms involved in obesity that could be used in different contexts. A general outline of one such approach is presented below. Williams (1984) has described another approach directed at characterizing morbid obesity and he discusses some of the issues of data collection not considered here.

A.   Defining the Trait

One of the first tasks that must be accomplished in any genetic or family study is to establish what trait will be studied. This sounds simple enough, but in the case of obesity it may be quite complex. What do we mean when we are talking about obesity or obesity-related traits? Do we mean overweight? And how is that defined? Is obesity simply a large body mass index (W/S^2)? Is it excess total body fat or a large percent body fat? Or is it a behavioral trait relating to increased appetite or decreased exercise? Should we be more focused and deal with an abnormal lipid level or an enzyme related to fat metabolism? The possibilities are almost endless and can go beyond individual measures to include traits such as the pattern of fat distribution on an individual at one point in time, or in serial data the patterns of change in a trait over time in an individual (e.g., adolescent versus adult onset, onset at pregnancy, etc.). It can be a syndrome (in the qualitative sense) or function of many separate measures (in the quantitative sense). Classical genetic studies have focused exclusively on qualitative traits, but as referenced above, over the past 10 to 15 years many analytical approaches have been developed to deal with quantitative traits.

The first step in studying the genetics of obesity is to choose an appropriate trait (or traits) for study. The more clearly defined the phenotype, the more likely specific mechanisms involved in the trait will be identified. Also, it is often argued that the closer the trait is to the biochemical process involved, the more likely specific genetic factors can be identified. As mentioned below, heterogeneity in a trait can severely complicate an analysis and obscure genetic mechanisms. Thus one area of research that should be addressed is the characterization (and categorization) of obesity in an epidemiological sense with concurrent emphasis on identifying biochemical mechanisms involved in the various types of obesity.

B. Establishing the Familial Nature of the Trait

Usually, determining that a trait is familial is not difficult and does not require very sophisticated methodologies. Clues are often obtained in population-based-epidemiological studies involving families, or from studies within ethnic groups. As reviewed above, traditional family studies of obesity-related traits have done little more than establish the familial nature of the trait. Research that only establishes that a trait is familial, should be discouraged. Examining the familial nature of new obesity-related traits as they are defined should be done in the context of larger more comprehensive studies.

C. Dealing with Problems Occurring in Family Studies

There are a number of problems faced in family studies of obesity. The heterogeneity in obesity-related traits is a major stumbling block. This heterogeneity relates to the likely variety of mechanisms leading to similar phenotypes (outcomes). Expressed in another way, it seems likely that there are a number of different types of obesity, and attempting to establish specific genetic mechanisms of high level traits such as total body fatness, body mass index, etc. in a population-based family study is likely to fail without some means of establishing more homogeneous subgroups of individuals (families) with the same type of obesity or appropriately dealing with heterogeneity in the analysis.

Another major problem in doing familial studies of obesity relates to the obvious influences of environmental factors. The higher the level (the more removed from the biochemical level) of the trait, the more opportunity it has to be influenced by environmental factors. Clearly, in the United States as well as other countries, there are strong sociocultural influences affecting the environment as it relates to obesity and the factors affecting body fatness. Obesity as a general trait is far from ideal for genetic studies. With respect to environmental influences another problem is the generational differences in environment and its effect on the trait, in other words, secular trends in the trait.

Finally, a problem that must be dealt with in virtually all family studies is age and sex variation in the trait. While these effects may be dealt with in a variety of ways, some more appropriate than others, they remain an important consideration in familial studies. Future research must address these problems seriously and deal with them in an analytically appropriate fashion.

D.   Dissecting Genetic and Environmental Influences

Clearly, there is a familial aggregation of body fatness, but the extent to which this is genetic is less certain. The recent work of Stunkard and colleagues (1986) suggests that genetic influences play a large and important role in the familial nature of adult age-sex adjusted body mass index. Other obesity-related traits may show similar or different results. Some studies indicate relatively little genetic involvement for subcutaneous fat thickness. Others indicate that lipids and lipoprotein levels, for example, show strong genetic determination. In some of our own data, familial correlations for W/S^2 and calf circumference change with age of the individuals involved in the correlations, indicating varying environmental involvement over time (Byard et al., 1983).

After determining that a trait is familial, the next step is to determine whether the familial nature of the trait results from genetic or environmental factors. Approaches to this question are many and include twin studies, adoption studies, studies of correlations between pairs of relatives, etc. Generally, the aim is to determine what portion of the variation in the trait is due to genetic factors, and what portion is due to environmental ones. Clearly, genetic factors play an important role, but few adequate genetic studies have been made.

In typical family studies social or cultural inheritance (behaviors, etc. that are passed among family members in a manner that can be confused with genetic transmission) may inflate estimates of genetic involvement. Path analysis, which is basically a complex regression analysis, is well suited for separating genetic and environmental variation and for estimating the degree of cultural inheritance (Elston and Rao, 1978; Cloninger et al., 1983). That is, path analysis including studies of adoptive families can help to separate genetic and cultural inheritance and provide better estimates of the true level of genetic involvement in a trait. Path analysis can not, however, be used to determine specific genetic mechanisms.

Future research should address the very important issue of dissecting random environmental effects from inherited factors involved in the variation of obesity-related traits. In addition, cultural inheritance should be separated from true genetic influences to understand more accurately the actual level of genetic involvement in the trait.

E.   Establishing the Genetic Mechanism

In terms of ultimate usefulness, it would be most desirable to identify single factors that have some influence on the trait. Thus, one logical approach to establishing the genetic mechanism is to look for major gene effects. For our purposes a major gene may be loosely defined as a single gene or gene complex that has a measurable (large) effect on the trait, that is, an appreciable portion of the variation in the trait results from a single gene. One reason for the interest in major gene effects is because of the relevance in terms of genetic counseling and treatment. A single gene implies a very specific biochemical defect. Mathematical functions of obesity-related variables may be used as a single trait in quantitative analysis, the rationale being that the combination of variables better identifies the pleiotropic effects of a single gene.

The analytical approaches to identifying specific genetic mechanisms are through segregation/pedigree analysis (Elston and Stewart, 1971; Morton, 1982; Bonney, 1984, 1986). These are complex statistical methodologies that allow the separation of effects of major genes, polygenes and environmental factors in relatively specific ways. In addition, they may provide evidence for specific dominance relationships between the alleles of the major gene. Depending on the specific approach being used, the family data may consist of a large number of nuclear families (parents and their children) or a smaller number of large pedigrees (50 to several hundred people). These methodologies require significant computer resources and a well-trained quantitative geneticist to perform and interpret. They have evolved over the past ten to fifteen years and provided one basis for the field of study that deals with the genetics of multifactorial diseases, the field of genetic epidemiology.

After identifying a major gene effect, it is of interest to determine the location of the gene on the human genetic map. This may be done with genetic linkage studies, in which known single gene genetic markers (e.g., blood groups, enzyme variants) are used to determine if the major gene is near one of the markers on a specific human chromosome (Ott, 1984).

Beyond these approaches newer biochemical and molecular genetic methodologies are providing additional tools to identify and map genes involved with multifactorial traits such as obesity. Currently there is high interest in using DNA restriction fragment length polymorphisms (RFLPs) in apolipoprotein research to help better understand the genetic mechanisms involved in atherosclerosis and early coronary artery disease. While they have been excluded from consideration in this presentation, animal models are very important tools that should be used and may help provide a better understanding of genetic factors operating in obesity.

Too often in the past, studies of obesity reporting genetic findings have not been specifically designed with genetic hypotheses in mind. That is, the genetic results are a by-product of a study designed for some other purpose. Future research should focus on elucidating genetic mechanisms for specific traits. Studies should be designed to employ appropriate genetic epidemiological methodologies that can provide information about the mechanisms involved. A new area that shows promise in some situations involves molecular biological methodologies applied in genetic epidemiological settings.

V. Summary and Recommendations for Future Study

Aims of future research should attempt to determine specific genetic mechanisms operating in fat-related traits. Some traits to be studied may result from a better characterization (and categorization) of obesity in a biological and epidemiological sense. Research that only establishes that a trait is familial should be discouraged. Examining the familial nature of new obesity-related traits as they are defined should be done in the context of larger, more comprehensive studies. Problems such as heterogeneity, environmental influences, secular trends, age and sex differences must be dealt with in an analytically appropriate fashion. Path analysis can be used to estimate cultural inheritance which must be separated from true genetic influences to characterize more accurately for the level of genetic involvement in the trait. The presence of genetic linkage between genes controlling specific fat measures and genetic markers, including RFLPs, should be investigated. Studies should be designed to employ appropriate genetic epidemiological methodologies that can provide information about the mechanisms involved.

References

Angel, J. L. (1949). Constitution in female obesity. *Am. J. Phys. Anthrop.*, 7:433–471.

Bauer, J. (1945). *Constitution and Disease* (2nd ed.). New York: Grune and Stratton.

Bonney, G. E. (1984). On the statistical determination of major gene mechanisms in continuous human traits: Regressive models. *Am. J. Med. Genet.*, 18:731–749.

Bonney, G. E. (1986). Regressive logistic models for familial disease and other binary traits. *Biometrics*, 42:611–626.

Bouchard, C., Demirjian, A. & Malina, R. (1980). Path analysis of family resemblance in physique. *Stud. Phys. Anthrop.*, 6:61–70.

Bouchard, C., Savard, R., Despres, J. P., Tremblay, A. & Leblanc, C. (1985). Body composition in adopted and biological siblings. *Hum. Biol.*, 57:61–75.

Boyle, C. R. & Elston, R. C. (1979). Multifactorial genetic models for quantitative traits in humans. *Biometrics*, 35:55–68.

Bray, G. A. (1984). Hypothalamic and genetic obesity: An appraisal of the autonomic hypothesis and the endocrine hypothesis. *Int. J. Obes.*, 8:(Suppl. 1)119–137.

Bray, G. A. & York, D. A. (1971). Genetically transmitted obesity in rodents. *Physiol. Rev.*, 51:598–646.

Bruch, H. (1957). The case for heredity. pp. 86–251. In *The Importance of Overweight*. New York: W. W. Norton.

Burt, C. (1966). The genetic determination of differences in intelligence. A study of monozygotic twins reared together and apart. *Brit. J. Psychol.*, *57*:137−153.

Byard, P. J., Siervogel, R. M. and Roche, A. F. (1983). Sibling correlations for weight/stature squared and calf circumference: Age changes and possible sex linkage. *Hum. Biol.*, *55*:677−686.

Clark, P. J. (1956). The heritability of certain anthropometric characters as ascertained from measurement of twins. *Am. J. Hum. Genet.*, *8*:49−54.

Cloninger, C. R., Rao, D. C., Rice, J., Reich, T. & Morton, N. E. (1983). A defense of path analysis in genetic epidemiology. *Am. J. Hum. Genet.*, *35*:733−756.

Curnow, R. N. & Smith, C. (1975). Multifactorial models for familial diseases in man (with discussion). *J. Roy. Stat. Soc. (Series A), 138*:131−169.

Davenport, C. B. (1923). *Body Build and Its Inheritance*. Washington, D.C.: Carnegie Institution.

Dunlop, D. M. & Lyon, R. M. M. (1931). A study of 523 cases of obesity. *Edinburgh Med. J., 38*:561−577.

Ellis, R. W. B. & Tallerman, K. H. (1934). Obesity in childhood. Study of 50 cases. *Lancet, ii*:615−620.

Elston, R. C. & Rao, D. C. (1978). Statistical modeling and analysis in human genetics. *Ann. Rev. Biophy. and Bio. Engl., 7*:253−286.

Elston, R. C. & Stewart, J. (1971). A general model for the genetic analysis of pedigree data. *Hum. Hered., 21*:523−542.

Feinleib, M., Garrison, R. J., Fabsitz, R., Christian, J. C., Hrubec, Z., Borhani, N. O., Kannel, W. B., Rosenman, R., Schwartz, J. T. & Wagner, J. P. (1977). The NHLBI twin study of cardiovascular disease risk factors: Methodology and summary of results. *Am. J. Epidemiol., 106*:284−295.

Fellows, H. H. (1931). Studies of relatively normal obese individuals during and after dietary restrictions. *Am. J. Med. Sci., 181*:301−312.

Garn, S. M., Clark, D. C. & Ullman, B. M. (1975). Does obesity have a genetic basis in man? *Ecology Food & Nutr., 4*:57−59.

Gordon, H. H. (1957). A summary of some clinical aspects of obesity. *Pediatrics, 20*: 556−560.

Greenwood, M. R., Cleary, M. P. & Hirsch, J. (1979). Genetic obesity in man and rodents. *Curr. Concepts Nutr., 8*:143−170.

Gurney, R. (1936). The hereditary factor in obesity. *Arch. Intern. Med., 57*:557−561.

Hanis, C. L., Sing, C. F., Clarke, W. R. & Schrott, H. G. (1983). Multivariate models for human genetic analysis: Aggregation, coaggregation, and tracking of systolic blood pressure and weight. *Am. J. Hum. Genet., 35*:1196−1210.

Hawk, L. J. & Brook, C. G. (1979). Family resemblances of height, weight and body fatness. *Arch. Dis. Child., 54*:877−879.

Heller, R., Garrison, R. J., Havlik, R. J., Feinleib, M. & Padgett, S. (1984). Family resemblances in height and relative weight in the Framingham Heart Study. *Int. J. Obes., 8*:399−405.

Iversen, T. (1953). Psychogenic obesity in children. *I. Acta Paediat., 42*:8−19.

Johnson, M. L., Burke, B. S. & Mayer, J. (1956). Relative importance of inactivity and overeating in energy balance of obese high school girls. *Am. J. Clin. Nutr., 4*:37−44.

Karlin, S., Williams, P. T., Jensen, S. & Farquhar, J. W. (1981). Genetic analysis of the Stanford LRC family study data. 1. Structured exploratory data analysis of height and weight measurements. *Am. J. Epidemiol., 113*:307−324.

Khoury, P., Morrison, J. A., Laskarzewski, P. M. & Glueck, C. J. (1983). Parent-offspring and sibling body mass index associations during and after sharing of common household environments: The Princeton School District Family Study. *Metabolism, 32*:82−89.

Lange, K., Westlake, J. & Spence, M. A. (1976). Extensions to pedigree analysis. III. Variance components by the scoring method. *Ann. Hum. Genet., 39*:485−491.

Mann, G. V. (1974). The influence of obesity on health, II. *New Engl. J. Med., 291*:226−232.

Martin, A. O., Kurczynski, T. W. & Steinberg, A. G. (1973). Familial studies of medical and anthropometric variables in a human isolate. *Am. J. Hum. Genet., 25*:581−593.

Matsuki, S. & Yoda, R. (1971). Familial occurrence of obesity. An observation about height and weight of college women and their parents. *Keio J. Med., 20*:135−141.

Matsuki, S., Yoda, R. & Kataoka, K. (1971). Obesity in the Japanese, its prevalence and major complications. *Keio J. Med., 20*:127−133.

Mayer, J. (1960). Genetic factors in obesity. *Bull. N. Y. Acad. Med., 36*:323−343.

Mayer, J. (1968). *Overweight. Causes, Cost, and Control.* Englewood Cliffs, N. J.: Prentice-Hall.

McKusick, V. A. (1975). *Mendelian Inheritance in Man.* (4th ed.) Baltimore: Johns Hopkins Press.

Morton, N. E. (1982). *Outline of Genetic Epidemiology.* New York: S. Karger.

Morton, N. E., Rao, D. C. & Lalouel, J. M. (1983). *Methods in Genetic Epidemiology.* New York: S. Karger.

Mossberg, H. O. (1948). Basal metabolism in obesity in children. *Nord. Med., 39*:1718−1720.

Mueller, W. H. (1983). The genetics of human fatness. *Yearbook Phys. Anthrop., 26*:15−230.

Mullins, A. G. (1958). The prognosis in juvenile obesity. *Arch. Dis. Child., 33*:307−314.

Newman, H. H., Freeman, F. N. & Holzinger, K. J. (1937). *Twins. A Study of Heredity and Environment.* Chicago: University of Chicago Press.

Osborne, R. H. & De George, F. V. (1959). *Genetic Basis of Morphological Variation. An Evaluation and Application of the Twin Study Method.* Cambridge: Harvard University Press.

Ott, J. (1984). *Analysis of Human Genetic Linkage.* Baltimore: Johns Hopkins University Press.

Rao, D. C., MacLean, C. J., Morton, N. E. & Yee, S. (1975). Analysis of family resemblance. V. Height and weight in northeastern Brazil. *Am. J. Hum. Genet., 27*:509−520.

Reynolds, E. L. (1951). The distribution of subcutaneous fat in childhood and adolescence. *Soc. Res. Child Develop. Monogr.,* Serial no. 50.

Romaniuk-Michalska, E. & Krotkiewski, M. (1969). Genetical aspects of obesity. *Pol. Arch. Med. Wewn., 42*:465−474.

Rona, R. J. (1981). Genetic and environmental factors in growth in childhood. *Br. Med. Bull. 37*:265−272.

Rony, H. R. (1940). Obesity and leanness. In *Hereditary vs. Environmental Factors in Obesity and Leanness.*(pp176−209). Philadelphia: Lea & Febiger.

Savard, R., Bouchard, C., Leblanc, C. & Tremblay, A. (1983). Familial resemblance in fatness indicators. *Ann. Hum. Biol., 10*:111−118.

Schulsinger, F. (1985). The experience from the adoption method in genetic research. *Prog. Clin. Biol. Res., 177*:461−478.

Seltzer, C. C. (1967). Genetic and anthropologic factors in obesity. *Mod. Treatm., 4*:1096−1110.

Seltzer, C. C. & Mayer, J. (1964). Body build and obesity. Who are the obese? *J. Am. Med. Assoc., 189*:677−684.

Shenker, I. R., Visichelli, V. & Lang, J. (1974). Weight differences between foster infants of overweight and nonoverweight foster mothers. *J. Pediat., 84*:715−719.

Steinberg, A. G. (1960). Comments on the genetics of human obesity. *Am. J. Clin. Nutr., 8*:752−759.

Stewart, A. W., Jackson, R. T., Ford, M. A. & Beaglehole, R. (1987). Underestimation of relative weight by use of self-reported height and weight. *Am. J. Epidemiol.*, *125*:122−126.

Stunkard, A. J., Sorensen, T. I., Hanis, C., Teasdale, T. W., Chakraborty, R., Schull, W. J. & Schulsinger, F. (1986). An adoption study of human obesity. *N. Engl. J. Med.*, *314*:193−198.

Tanner, J. M. (1955). Obesity and classification of body build. *Advancement in Sci.*, *12*:116−120.

Thompson, E. A. (1985). *Pedigree analysis in human genetics*. Baltimore: Johns Hopkins University Press.

Trayhurn, P. (1984). The development of obesity in animals: The role of genetic susceptibility. *Clin. Endocrinol. Metab.*, *13*:451−474.

Vamberova, M., Prchlikova, H., Ticha, H. & Cerny, M. (1968). Genealogicke aspekty obezity. *Cs. Pediat.* (Praha), *25*:497−502.

Von Verschuer, O. (1927). Die vererbungsbiologische Zwillingsforschung. *Ergeb. Inn. Med. Kindh.*, *31*:35−120.

Williams, R. R. (1984). The role of genetic analyses in characterizing obesity. *Int. J. Obes.*, *8*:551−559.

Withers, R. F. J. (1961). A genetical study of human obesity. *2nd Int. Congr. Hum. Genet.*, Rome. *2*:1058−1063.

Withers, R. F. J. (1964). Problems in the genetics of human obesity. *Eugen. Rev.*, *56*:81−90.

4

Does Early Eating Behavior Influence Later Adiposity?

W. STEWART AGRAS
Stanford University School of Medicine
Stanford, California

The recent National Institutes of Health consensus panel on the health implications of obesity noted that any degree of overweight may be associated with an increased health risk. They recommended that everyone who is more than 20% overweight should reduce, and urged more research aimed at preventing this widespread disorder of modern living (National Institutes of Health, 1985). Among the necessary conditions for the successful prevention of obesity are a means of identifying the infant or child at high risk of developing obesity in later life; the identification of remediable risk factors; and an effective intervention program. While the prevention of this problematic disorder may be many years away, it is almost certain that early childhood will be an important arena for such efforts, for the long-term results of the treatment of obesity are often disappointing both in adults and in children (Weil, 1977). Moreover, infancy and early childhood would appear to be a critical period during which fat cells are developed (Knittle, Timmers, Ginsberg-Fellner, Brown, & Katz, 1979). Thus, it is important to delineate the remediable factors influencing such development. This chapter will review the evidence for the existence of one class of potential risk factors for obesity, namely the characteristics of early feeding behavior that may be associated with the development of later adiposity, discuss the clinical implications of the findings to date, and consider the research steps necessary to further advance our understanding of this class of risk factors.

I. Caloric Intake and Early Adiposity

At first thought it seems remarkable that there is controversy over the relationship between caloric intake during infancy and either concurrent or later adiposity. However, measurement of the energy intake of infants is by no means easy, and different methods have been used in different studies, including: maternal reports of their infants' intake; weighing infants before and after feedings; weighing formula and food intakes (for those not being breastfed); and determining the amount and characteristics of expressed breast milk. Each of these methods has its problems. Thus, the error of measurement, which differs from method to method, varies from study to study. In addition, many of the studies of the relationship between the caloric intake and adiposity in infancy have small sample sizes. Thus, the power of such studies is small, and the representativeness of the sample questionable. In addition, measures of adiposity vary. Some studies use weight, which is not a good measure of adiposity since it includes both lean body mass and fat; other studies use skinfold thickness, which has a large error of measurement; and still others use various mathematically derived indices of adiposity such as Body Mass Index (BMI = W/H^2). It is not surprising, then, that there is conflicting evidence concerning the influence of caloric intake on adiposity in infants, and that some studies demonstrate a relationship between caloric intake and measures of adiposity while others do not.

Three lines of evidence do, however, suggest that there is a relationship between caloric intake and adiposity in infancy. These include studies of the relationship between measures of energy intake and adiposity; the relationship between weight gain in infancy and later adiposity; and the relationship between the type of feeding and later adiposity. Typical of the studies demonstrating a relationship between caloric intake and adiposity, Dewey and Lonnerdal (1983) studied 20 breast-fed infants over the first six months of life, collecting 24-hour records of infant food intake from mothers, and also analyzing a breast milk sample. Estimated caloric intake was significantly correlated with weight-for-length (r = 0.51) at two months of age, but not at four or six months of age. However, average energy intake over the first six months of life was significantly correlated with both weight gain during the first six months, and weight for length at six months of age. Cross-cultural comparisons also suggest that caloric intake is an important determinant of obesity. Thus, a British sample of infants took in significantly more calories than a comparable Swedish sample and demonstrated twice the prevalence of overweight compared to the Swedish sample (Sveger, Lindberg, Weibull, and Olsson, 1975). On the other hand, a study of 450 children from the age of six months to nine years, in which three-day food records were collected from mothers revealed little evidence for a relationship between caloric intake and adiposity at any age (Shapiro, Crawford, Clark, Pearson, Raz, and Huenemann, 1984).

A.   Rate of Weight Gain and Adiposity

The second line of evidence relating caloric intake to adiposity depends on the observed relationship between the rate of weight gain in infancy and later measures of adiposity. Mellbin and Vuille (1973) found that the rate of weight gain during the first year of life was the most powerful factor predicting adiposity at seven years of age in both boys and girls. In another study the same authors (Mellbin and Vuille, 1976a) found that weight gain to above the 90th percentile in the first year of life was associated with a relative risk of obesity at seven years of age of 3.3 in males, and 1.7 in females. Presumably rapid weight gain during infancy is related to excessive caloric intake as noted above (Dewey and Lonnerdal, 1983). Moreover, there is some evidence that birth weight doubling time is now more rapid than it was in the past, perhaps due to better nutrition during infancy (Neumann and Alpaugh 1976). In addition, bottle-fed infants double their weight earlier than breast fed infants (Neumann and Alpaugh, 1976), and there is evidence that bottle feeding results in a greater caloric intake than breast feeding (Hovlander, Hagman, Hillervik, and Sjolin, 1982).

B.   Mode of Feeding and Adiposity

The third line of evidence suggests that mode of feeding is an important determinant of adiposity, although again the evidence is mixed. Once more, there are many methodologic difficulties in determining mode of feeding, for infants are often fed both by breast and bottle. Bottle-fed infants also tend to be fed solid foods at an earlier time than breast-fed infants, thus it is a pattern of feeding rather than a simple difference between breast or bottle feeding that is usually being assessed. Moreover, since the choice of feeding cannot be assigned at random, the breast/bottle comparison is inevitably confounded by other variables such as social class. Nonetheless, the majority of studies suggest that the bottle-fed infant gains weight more rapidly than the breast-fed infant (Fomon, Thomas, Filer, Ziegler, and Leonard, 1970), and tends to take in more calories than the breast-fed infant (Hovlander et al. 1982). Most of these studies do not control for variables such as maternal age, race, and socioeconomic status. However, one study that did, found a significant long-term protective effect of breast feeding (Kramer 1981). A prospective study of 462 healthy infants followed for two years found that breast feeding and the delayed introduction of solid foods exerted a protective effect against excess adiposity up to two years of age (Kramer, Barr, Leduc, Boisjoly, McVey-White, and Pless, 1985; Kramer, Barr, Leduc, Boisjoly, and Pless, 1985). This study, using multiple regression analyses again controlled for socioeconomic factors thus revealing the independent effect of mode of feeding on adiposity. Again, however, there have been studies that have not found any difference between breast- and bottle-fed infants in terms of the development of adiposity (eg. Dine, Gartside, Glueck, Rheines, Greene, and Khoury, 1979).

Taking all these lines of inquiry into account, we can conclude that there is reasonable evidence that caloric intake is related to the development of adiposity during infancy and early childhood, although other factors such as birthweight and activity levels may also be important determinants of later adiposity (Dewey and Lonnerdal, 1983; Mellbin and Vuille, 1973). Caloric intake during infancy is of course, the result of a complex interaction between mother and infant, each of whom plays a part in determining the daily energy intake of the baby. Thus it has been hypothesized that bottle feeding is more under maternal control than is breast feeding, and that, therefore, the tendency would be to overfeed the bottle-fed infant, i.e., to continue feeding until the bottle is empty. In line with this argument, as we have seen, is the observation that the bottle-fed infant consumes more calories than the breast-fed infant (Hovlander et al, 1982; Kohler, Meeuwise, and Mortensson, 1984). One determinant of the caloric intake of infants may be maternal preferences for a thin or chubby child. This preference was measured in a recent study (Kramer, Barr, Leduc, Boisjoly, and Pless, 1983) by having mothers of young infants indicate their preference for a series of line drawings of babies differing only in fatness. Older mothers of higher social class tended to prefer thinner babies. In addition, breast feeding mothers preferred thinner babies than did mothers who used bottle feeding. While this study does not reveal the behaviors by which mothers vary the caloric intakes of their infants, it does provide strong support for the notion that infant caloric intake is determined in part by maternal views about the way their infants should look.

Thus a set of inter-related parental factors are associated with the development of infant adiposity. These include a lower socioeconomic status and younger maternal age, and a maternal preference for a chubbier baby; these factors are associated in turn with a tendency to bottle feed rather than breast feed. Moreover, bottle feeding is associated with a tendency to introduce solid foods earlier, thus adding a further caloric load to the infant's diet.

II. Infant Feeding Behavior and Adiposity

While the energy intake of infants is partially under maternal control, the feeding interaction is reciprocal. What part, then, does the infant play in determining caloric intake? Stylistic differences in early feeding behavior may well play an important role.

A. Feeding Style

It has long been suspected that obese individuals may differ in eating style from thinner individuals, although there are major methodological difficulties to overcome in the measurement of eating style. Measures have for the most part been observational, but the situation in which the measures have been made varies from the laboratory to the natural environment. Whether or not the subject knows that he is being observed is also an important variable, possibly affecting the obese more than the non-obese. The type of food being eaten is also important, for food that is difficult to chew will be eaten less rapidly than food that is easy to chew. Variation in food choices between the obese and non-obese could easily confound the measurement of eating style. Direct observational studies of eating behavior do, however, suggest that there is a difference between the eating behavior of obese and non-obese children. In one study, 30 overweight and 30 normal-weight preschool children were observed eating a lunch at school (Drabman, Cordua, Hammer, Jarvie, and Horton, 1979). At each age from 18 months to 7 years and older, the obese children ate more rapidly, as measured by the number of bites taken in each 30-second interval, than did the normal children. In addition, the overweight were found to chew their food less.

These findings in children have been echoed in studies of adults. In one study, obese women were found to eat more rapidly and to chew their food less than thin women (Adams, Ferguson, Stunkard, and Agras, 1978). In addition, replicating the findings from laboratory studies (Meyer and Pudel, 1977), the obese women did not slow down their eating, as measured by chewing rate, as the meal progressed, while the thin and normal weight women did. Other studies have found similar differences between obese and normal-weight individuals (Gaul, Craighead, and Mahoney, 1975; Marston, London, Cohen and Cooper, 1976), but again there have been studies that have found no differences (Dodd, Birky, and Stalling, 1976; Rosenthal and Marx, 1978; Warner and Balagura, 1975).

Turning to infancy, it has been found that heavier newborns tend to suck significantly more rapidly and consume significantly more formula if it is sweetened, than do lighter infants (Engen, Lipsitt, and Robinson,

1968; Nisbett and Gurwitz, 1974). The persistence of such behavior and food preferences through infancy would inevitably lead to a greater overall caloric intake and to fatter infants and children. These findings were expanded upon in a more recent study in which suckling rate and pressure of suckling were studied while controlling for intake, thus providing a measure of avidity of feeding (Milstein, 1980). Babies of medium or greater adiposity indeed showed a greater avidity for sweet-tasting fluids than did thinner babies. Thin babies, however, demonstrated a relative aversion for the sweet taste, suggesting a protective influence of thinness. This behavior pattern was found to predict relative weight at three years of age.

Overall, there is a reasonable body of evidence stretching from early infancy to adult life, suggesting that the obese exhibit a more vigorous eating style, or that, conversely, the thin demonstrate a less vigorous style.

B.   Suckling behavior

Most of the work in infancy is, however, based upon concurrent measures of feeding behavior and adiposity. Thus it is not possible to determine the direction of influence. Is it that the heavy child at birth has a more vigorous eating style? Or does an avid feeding style influence later adiposity? This question was recently addressed in a study from our laboratory (Agras, Kraemer, Berkowitz, Korner, and Hammer 1987). To measure the style of infant suckling, as well as caloric intake from a particular feeding, infants were brought into the laboratory at two and four weeks of age. In earlier work, Kron and his colleagues (Kron, Ipsen, and Goddard, 1968) had developed a method of recording the fine detail of infant sucking behavior, using an apparatus referred to as a suckometer. This apparatus consists of a constant pressure reservoir containing formula connected by a rigid nipple held within an ordinary nursing bottle by noncollapsible tubing. A pressure transducer connected to a side arm allows recording of the feed upon a polygraph. At each of the feeds in our study, the mother fed the infant while sitting comfortably. Adiposity in this study was measured by skinfold thickness at 1 and 2 years of age.

The univariate relationships between the major measures of interest and infant adiposity at one and two years of age are shown in Table 1. As can be seen, the main relationships of interest are between variables describing the infants' feeding pattern (sucking pressure, interburst interval, and number of feeds/day) and adiposity. In addition, parental education is weakly related to triceps skinfold thickness at one year of age. Note that caloric intake is not significantly related to adiposity in childhood.

Table I

Univariate correlations between the major potential predictor variables and triceps skinfold thickness at 1 and 2 years of age

	Triceps 1 yr	Triceps 2 yrs
Triceps 2 wks	−.041	−.079
Father's triceps	−0.080	−.139
Mother's triceps	.099	.085
Parental education	−.182+	−.102
Caloric intake	.034	.186
Duration breast feeding	0.12	.125
Number of feeds/day	−.143	−.235*
Sucking pressure	.157	.290**
Interburst interval	−0.199*	−.214*

$^+ p < .1$ $^* p < .05$ $^{**} p < .01$

The results of a multiple regression analysis using the variables listed in Table 1, and conducted separately for skinfold thickness at one and two years of age, are shown in Table 2. At one year of age the combination of educational level of the parents and interburst interval explains some 18% of the variance in skinfold thickness, while at two years of age, the pressure of suckling and number of feeds per day explains some 21% of the variance.

Thus feeding behaviors, particularly early suckling, appear to determine adiposity as measured by skinfold thickness at both one and two years of age. What kind of suckling pattern characterizes the infant who is likely to be a fatter child? To answer this question, the variables demonstrating

Table 2

Multiple Regression analyses for skinfold thickness at 1 and 2 years of age

Skinfold thickness 1 year (n = 81)		
Factor	Multiple $r2$	P
Education	−0.105	<0.004
Interburst interval	−0.182	<0.02
Skinfold thickness 2 years (n = 79)		
Factor	Multiple $r2$	P
Pressure of suckling	0.134	<0.006
Number of feeds/day	0.214	<0.01

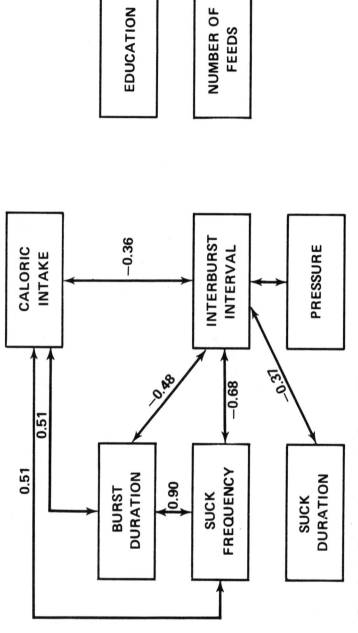

Figure 1. A diagram demonstrating the correlations of suckling characteristics with the predictors of adiposity at 1 and 2 years of age, and with caloric intake.

a significant correlation with pressure and interburst interval are displayed in Figure 1. As can be seen, interburst interval is negatively correlated with pressure of suckling and with suck frequency, which in turn is correlated with burst duration. Both interburst interval and suck frequency are correlated with caloric intake. Thus an infant who sucks more frequently at a higher pressure, with short intervals between long bursts of sucking, will tend to take in more calories and will also tend to be fatter. A typical example of a vigorous feeding style is compared with a less vigorous style in Figure 2. The very early appearance of a distinctive pattern of suckling associated with adiposity suggests that such a pattern is inborn rather than learned. Indeed, it is possible that this behavior pattern is an expression of the genetic tendency toward obesity. Infants with a genetic tendency toward the development of obesity may demonstrate this vigorous pattern of suckling.

The other factors associated with a tendency toward the development of adiposity in childhood are the number of feeds per day during the first five months of life, and parental educational level. The number of feeds per day was negatively related to the degree of adiposity in childhood. Number of feeds per day was also negatively correlated with caloric intake during laboratory suckling ($r = 0.25$, $p < .01$). Thus, the vigorously feeding infant takes in more calories with each feed than the less vigorous feeder. Animal studies have repeatedly demonstrated an inverse relationship between number of feeds per day and adiposity, suggesting that the patterning of feeds affects energy intake. The relationship between parental educational level and adiposity was such that the higher the parents educational attainment, the thinner the child was likely to be. This finding is in accord with other epidemiologic evidence implicating social class level as an important determinant of obesity (Stunkard 1986). As noted earlier in this chapter, mothers of higher social class demonstrate a preference for a thinner looking baby (Kramer et al, 1983). The mechanism by which such mothers influence their infants weight is not known, although several possibilities are apparent. First, it is possible that parents with a higher educational level are less likely to be genetically predisposed to develop obesity, and would thus tend to have thin infants. It has been shown, for example, that obese individuals tend to be selected against when applying to college, despite equal intelligence. This in turn would tend to lower future socioeconomic status. Second, it is possible that such mothers tend to feed their infants fewer calories, perhaps substituting other activities with their infants for feeding. Along the same lines, parents with higher educational levels may stimulate their children more, thus inducing higher levels of activity and protecting against the excessive development of adiposity.

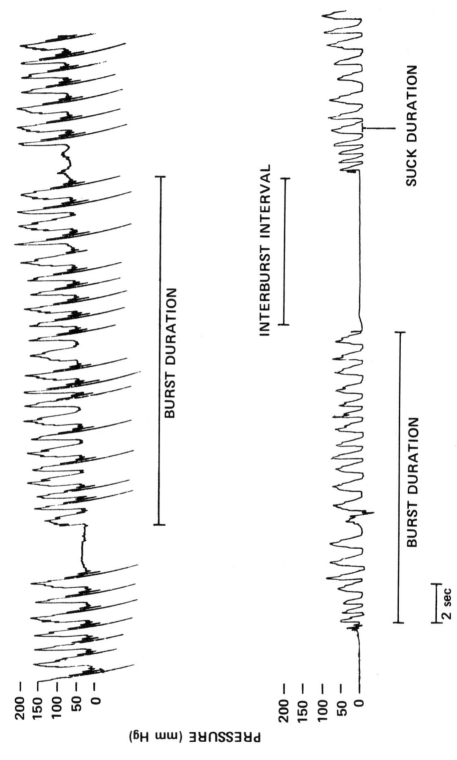

Figure 2. A tracing from two infants with contrasting feeding styles. The upper tracing shows an infant with a vigorous feeding style (high pressure, short interburst interval, long burst duration, and rapid suckling) while the lower tracing is from an infant less vigorous

C.   Do Fat Babies Remain Fat?

As noted at the beginning of this chapter, in order to prevent obesity by intervening at an early age, it is necessary to identify risk factors that predict the occurrence of obesity in later years, preferably in adult life when the effects of obesity upon health become more apparent. Thus it is important to determine how well measures of adiposity are related to one another over the years. It has been shown that the chubby infant has an increased risk of becoming an overweight child (Mack and Johnston, 1976; Mellbin and Vuille, 1976), or even an obese adult (Charney, Goodman, McBride, Lyon, and Pratt, 1976), a relative risk that varies between 2:1 and 4:1 depending upon the sample studied and the length of follow-up. Unfortunately, low risk ratios of this sort suggest that identifying which child will become obese on the basis of early adiposity will lead to a high proportion of both false positive and false negative tests. Garn and Lavelle (1985) have shown that about one-quarter of obese infants will remain obese two decades later. Charney et al (1976) found that 36% of infants at or above the 90th percentile in weight for height would become either obese or overweight adults. Other potential indicators of future obesity in infancy, such as birth weight, and the rate of weight increase during the first six months of life, are only weakly associated with later adiposity (Eid, 1970; Mellbin and Vuille, 1976b; Shapiro et al, 1984;) and hence are also not useful predictors. The addition of information concerning the relative weight of the parents does, however, somewhat improve predictive power (Garn, Bailey, and Solomon, 1981).

New light was recently shed on the problem of prediction of obesity by a group of French researchers who examined the development of adiposity, as measured by BMI, from infancy to adolescence (Rolland-Cachera, Deheeger, Bellisle, Sempe, Guillod-Bataille, and Patois, 1984). These workers found that BMI peaked during the first year of life and thereafter fell, only to rise once more between the ages of five and ten years, changes that appear to reflect the course of fat cell development (Knittle et al. 1979). An example of this developmental curve for a cohort of adolescents followed from birth to 14 years of age is shown in Figure 3. The process of development of adiposity from birth to 14 years for the group as a whole is depicted as the center curve. As noted by Rolland-Cachera et al. (1984), adiposity (as measured by BMI) increases sharply during the first year of life, demonstrating an initial peak at about the age of one year, and then declines for several years until, after reaching a low point (referred to as the trough), it once more increases. The difference in the development of BMI between the group who became obese in adolescence, and those remaining at normal weight is shown by the upper and lower curves in Figure 3. The group that will become obese tends to

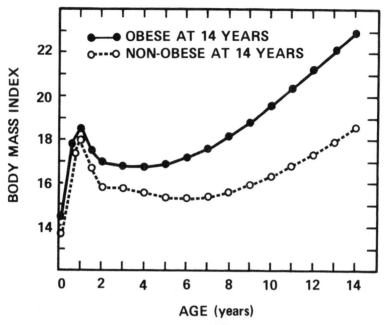

Figure 3. The development of adiposity from birth to 14 years of age in a cohort of infants who will be obese in adolescence (upper curve) and who will be of normal weight (lower curve). Those who will become obese are slightly more adipose at birth and at the 1 year peak, lose less fat during the second year of life, and demonstrate an earlier increase in adiposity than those who will be normal weight at 14 years.

be slightly heavier at birth than those who will remain thin, reaches a higher peak BMI slightly later in infancy (BMI=22.9 at 14.1 months vs BMI=21.6 at 12.0 months), and shows less decline in BMI at about the age of two years. The major difference between the two groups begins in the fourth year of life with an earlier rise in BMI for those who will become obese (50.0 months vs 70.4 months). The difference in mean weight between the two groups is 4.3 kg at five years of age, and 11.5 kg at 14 years of age.

It is likely that the decline in adiposity in the second year of life is associated with a decrease in adipocyte size, and that the increase in adiposity later in childhood is associated with an increase in fat cell number and size. This increase occurs earlier for the obese than for the non-obese. Children with a relatively large BMI at one year, who demonstrate an early rise in BMI level, tend to be obese in adolescence, while those with a low BMI at one year or a delayed rise, remained thin. It is possible that the addition of information concerning the age at which an increase in adiposity occurs would also increase the accuracy with which predictions might be made about future adiposity. Unfortunately, no data for the relative risk of developing obesity using this new factor are available.

It seems then, that there are at least two critical periods for the development of adiposity, the first during infancy associated with the factors described above, and the second during childhood at about four years of age for the obese, and later for those who will remain or become thin. While genetic factors are likely to loom large in these developments, the exact mechanism responsible for this second increase in adiposity is at present unknown. The existence of two critical periods for the development of adiposity, presumably governed by different mechanisms and affecting different individuals, would begin to explain why the correlation between measures of adiposity during infancy and childhood tend to be low, and why our ability to predict the development of obesity on the basis of infant adiposity is correspondingly poor.

D.   Some Further Discontinuities

A recent long-term follow-up study of a cohort of infants demonstrated that formula-fed infants were more adipose by 112 days, as measured by BMI, than were breast-fed infants (Fomon, Rogers, Ziegler, Nelson, and Thomas, 1984). There was no evidence, however, that the type of feeding during infancy influenced measures of adiposity at eight years of age. Cholesterol levels at eight years of age also showed no relationship to the mode of feeding during infancy. One interpretation of these data is that mode of feeding during infancy is not a critical factor in the longer term, and that other factors occurring either in infancy or later in childhood override the effects of breast or bottle feeding.

Yet another discontinuity in feeding behaviors was revealed recently in our laboratory (Berkowitz, Agras, Kraemer, and Korner). In this study, sucking behavior was measured in the laboratory at two and four weeks of age, and solid eating behaviors were observed in the same cohort at 18 months of age. If feeding behaviors were a continuum, with the vigorous suckling style developing into the obese rapid eating style, we would have expected to find that suckling and solid eating behaviors were related to one another. The suckling behaviors chosen for analysis were pressure, burst duration, active feed time, and caloric intake; while the solid eating behaviors were bite frequency, active feed time, the volume of liquids consumed, and caloric intake. No significant correlation was found between the sucking and solid eating behaviors, suggesting that these two sets of feeding behaviors are unrelated.

This finding replicates work in animals. Thus amphetamine diminishes food intake during solid eating in adult animals (Campbell, Lytle, and Fibiger, 1969). On the other hand, amphetamine increases the amount of time that rats suckle and does not decrease the amount of milk consumed (Williams and Brake, 1982). The weanling rat will both suckle and eat solid food depending on the feeding situation. It has been shown that when serotonin was blocked with methysergide in these young animals, weanling rats will suckle rather than eat solid food, even though nutritional deprivation caused little suckling in these animals (Williams, Hall, and Rosenblatt, 1979). When these animals were treated with a serotonin receptor agonist they began to eat solid food once again. Again these findings suggest that suckling and solid eating behavior are controlled by different neurochemical pathways. Interestingly, in contrast with the effects of amphetamine, serotonin blockade has little effect on the feeding behavior of the adult rat (Blundell, 1977).

Taken together with the developmental curve of adiposity described by Rolland-Cachera et al. (1984), these findings confirm the existence of discontinuities in the development of feeding behavior in infancy and childhood. The existence of such discontinuities enhances our understanding as to why adiposity does not track better across the early years of life and into adolescence.

III. Implications for Clinical Practice

One of the main problems delineated by the above discussion is the lack of well-identified risk factors in infancy that predict the later development of obesity. Perhaps the main implication for the clinician is that excessive adiposity in infancy should be treated conservatively. Even though the long-term effects of mode of feeding are uncertain, it seems reasonable to continue to promote the use of breast feeding and to delay the introduction of solid foods, for these modes of feeding have been shown in many, but not all studies, to protect against the development of excessive adiposity in infancy and early childhood. More frequent smaller feedings may provide additional protection against the development of excess adiposity.

The child most at risk to develop excessive adiposity will be one with a genetic predisposition toward the development of obesity, as revealed by a familial history of obesity. Such children will also have a higher relative weight at birth, and will demonstrate the vigorous feeding style described earlier in this chapter. Whether or not such a style of feeding is recognizable outside the laboratory remains to be seen, but it is not unlikely that mothers would recognize such a style of suckling. Whether or not the clinician should counsel such parents to avoid overfeeding their infant should probably await replication and extension of the present findings.

Relatively little work has been done to examine the effects of dietary intervention in infancy. Thus, there is little solid evidence on the efficacy and safety of dietary changes to guide the clinician. In one uncontrolled study, a diet relatively low in fat was prescribed for a cohort of infants (Pisacano, Lichter, Ritter, and Siegal, 1978). Only one of these infants became overweight by three years of age as compared with a prevalence of over 25% overweight in infants receiving a regular diet in the same practice. These findings are encouraging and provide some guidance for dietary intervention in the infant at high risk for the development of adiposity.

IV. Implications for Future Research

A number of risk factors associated with the development of adiposity in infancy and early childhood have now been identified including: Genetic predisposition, social class, maternal desire for a chubby infant, bottle feeding, early introduction of solid foods, less frequent feeding, a vigorous feeding style, an avidity for sweet fluids, and fewer feeds. Some of the relationships between these factors are presently unknown, and the exact contribution of each of these factors to later adiposity has not been worked out. Longitudinal studies of cohorts of infants to at least five years of age, when those who will show an early rise in adiposity will have been identified, are needed to clarify these issues.

Research to date has focused largely on the gain in adiposity during infancy and early childhood. An equally important, but entirely neglected area of research, is to identify the factors associated with the decline in adiposity during the second year of life, for the child who will remain obese will show less decline than the child who will become thin. In addition, the factors associated with the relatively early rise in adiposity during later childhood, a rise that characterizes those who will become obese children and adolescents, need to be clarified. Again, longitudinal studies of cohorts of infants and children are needed to examine these questions.

The various discontinuities noted between infancy and childhood in respect to the development of adiposity, the problems of early identification of infants at high risk of developing obesity as adults, and the possible risks associated with early dietary intervention, all suggest that infancy is not the ideal time for early intervention or prevention of obesity. On the other hand, considering the development curve of adiposity shown in Figure 3, it would seem that a primary prevention program should be in place before four years of age, the time at which the adiposity curve of the child who will become obese departs from that of the child who will remain or become thin. The aim of such a program would be to prolong troughing (i.e., to keep the child thinner for longer). Thus the time at which to begin a prevention program for obesity would seem to be between two and three years of age. Thus, interventions aimed at prolonging troughing need to be devised and tested, for this seems to be the critical effect needed to prevent the development of obesity. The characteristics of such a prevention program are mandated to some extent by our modest ability to predict which child will become an obese adult or adolescent. It is unlikely that more than one-half of a "high risk sample" of children with all the known risk factors would become obese in adolescence. Thus a prevention program must be relatively inexpensive, should have no deleterious effects, and should benefit those who will not become obese. While the characteristics of such a program are beyond the scope of this chapter, a heart-healthy diet with a relatively low fat content combined with increased activity and perhaps less television watching (Dietz, 1985) might be appropriate.

Steady progress has been made in the past 20 years in delineating some of the risk factors for obesity in infancy. Given the various problems of predicting forward from infancy, it seems that high priority should now be given to understanding the risk factors for obesity in early childhood. This is an area that has been neglected until now, yet the research findings presently available suggest that it may be a most fruitful arena for basic and applied biobehavioral studies.

References

Adams, N., Ferguson, J., Stunkard, A. J., & Agras, W. S. (1978). The eating behavior of obese and nonobese women. *Behaviour Research & Therapy, 16*, 225–232.

Berkowitz, R. I., Agras, W. S., Kraemer, H. C., & Korner, A. F. Human sucking and solid eating behaviors are unrelated.

Blundell, J. E. (1977). Is there a role for serotonin (5-hydroxytryptamine) in feeding? *International Journal of Obesity, 1*, 15–42.

Campbell, B. A., Lytle, L. D., & Fibiger, H. C. (1969). Ontogeny of adrenergic arousal and cholinergic inhibitory mechanisms in the rat. *Science, 166*, 635–637.

Charney, E., Goodman, H. C., McBride, M., Lyon, B., & Pratt, R. (1976). Childhood antecedents of adult obesity: Do chubby infants become obese adults? *New England Journal of Medicine, 295*, 6–9.

Dewey, K. G., & Lonnerdal, B. (1983). Milk and nutrient intake of breast fed infants from 1 to 6 months: Relation to growth and fatness. *Journal of Pediatric Gastroenterology and Nutrition, 2*, 497–506.

Dine, M. S., Gartside, P. S., Glueck, C. J., Rheines, L., Greene, G., & Khoury, P. (1979). Where do the heaviest infants come from? A prospective study of white children from birth to 5 years of age. *Pediatrics, 63*, 1–7.

Dietz, W. H., & Gortmaker, S. L. (1985). Do we fatten our children at the television set? Obesity and television viewing in children and adolescents. *Pediatrics, 75*, 807–812.

Dodd, D. K., Birky, H. J., & Stalling, R. B. (1976). Eating behavior of obese and nonobese females in a natural setting. *Addictive Behaviors, 2*, 321–325.

Drabman, R. S., Cordua, G. D., Hammer D., Jarvie, G. J., & Horton, W. (1979). Developmental trends in eating rates of normal and overweight preschool children. *Child Development, 50*, 211–216.

Eid, E. E. (1970). Follow-up study of physical growth of children who had excessive weight gain in first six months of life. *British Medical Journal, 2*, 74–76.

Engen, T., Lipsitt, L. P., Robinson, D. O. (1978). The human newborn's sucking behavior for sweet fluids as a function of birthweight and maternal weight. *Infant Behavior and Development, 1*, 118–121.

Fomon, S. J., Rogers, R. R., Ziegler, E. E., Nelson, S. E., & Thomas, L. N. (1984). Indices of fatness and serum cholesterol at age 8 years in relation to feeding and growth during early infancy. *Pediatric Research, 18*, 1233–1238.

Fomon, S. J., Thomas, L. N., Filer, L. J., Ziegler, E. E., & Leonard, M. T. (1971). Food consumption and growth of normal infants fed milk-based formulas. *Acta Paediatrica Scandinavica, 60*, 223–240.

Gaul, D. J., Craighead, W. E., & Mahoney, M. J. (1975). Relationship between eating rates and obesity. *Journal of Consulting and Clinical Psychology, 43*, 123–125.

Garn, S. M., Bailey, S. M., & Solomon, M. A. (1981). Effect of remaining family members on fatness prediction. *American Journal of Clinical Nutrition, 34*, 148–153.

Garn, S. M., & Lavelle, M. (1985). Two-decade follow-up of fatness in early childhood, *American Journal of Diseases of Children, 139*, 181–185.

Hofvander, Y., Hagman, U., Hillervik, C., & Sjolin, S. (1982). The amount of milk consumed by 1–2 months old breast- or bottle-fed infants. *Acta Paediatrica Scandinavica, 71*, 953–962.

Knittle, J. L., Timmers, K., Ginsberg-Fellner, F., Brown, R. E., & Katz, D. P. (1979). The growth of adipose tissue in children and adolescents: Cross-sectional and longitudinal studies of adipose cell number and size. *Journal of Clinical Investigation, 63*, 239–246.

Kohler, L., Meeuwise, G., & Mortensson, W. (1984). Food intake and growth of infants between 6 and 26 weeks of age on breast milk, cow's milk formula, or soy formula. *Acta Paediatrica Scandinavica, 73*, 40-48.

Kramer, M. S. (1981). Do breast-feeding and delayed introduction of solid foods protect against subsequent obesity? *Journal of Pediatrics, 98*, 883–887.

Kramer, M. S., Barr, R. G., Leduc, D. G., Boisjoly, C., & Pless, I. B. (1983). Maternal psychological determinants of infant obesity: Development and testing of 2 new instruments. *Journal of Chronic Disease, 4*, 329–333.

Kramer, M. S., Barr, R. G., Leduc, G., Boisjoly, C., McVey-White, L., & Pless, B. (1985). Determinants of weight and adiposity in the first year of life. *Journal of Pediatrics, 106*, 10–14.

Kramer, M. S., Barr, R. G., Leduc, D. G., Boisjoly, C., & Pless, B. (1985). Infant determinants of childhood weight and adiposity. *Journal of Pediatrics, 107*, 104–107.

Kron, R. E., Ipsen, J., & Goddard, K. E. (1968). Consistent individual differences in the nutritive sucking behavior of the human newborn. *Psychosomatic Medicine, 30*, 151–157.

Mack, R. W., & Johnston, F. E. (1976). The relationship between growth in infancy and growth in adolescence: Report of a longitudinal study among urban black adolescents. *Human Biology, 48,* 693–711.

Marston, A. R., London, P., Cohen, N., & Cooper, L. M. (1977). In vivo observation of the eating behavior of obese and non-obese subjects. *Journal of Consulting and Clinical Psychology, 45,* 335–336.

Mellbin, T., & Vuille, J. C. (1973). Physical development at 7 years of age in relation to velocity of weight gain in infancy with special reference to incidence of overweight. *British Journal of Preventative and Social Medicine, 27,* 225–235.

Mellbin, T., & Vuille, J. C. (1976a). The relative importance of rapid weight gain in infancy as a precursor of childhood obesity. *Pediatric Adolescence and Endocrine, 1,* 78–83.

Mellbin, T., & Vuille, J. C. (1976b). Relationship of weight gain in infancy to subcutaneous fat and relative weight at 10 1/2 years of age. *British Journal of Preventive and Social Medicine, 30,* 239–243.

Meyer, J. E. & Pudel, V. E. (1977). Experimental feeding in man: A behavioral approach to obesity. *Psychosomatic Medicine, 29,* 153–157.

Neumann, C. G., & Alpaugh, M. (1976). Birthweight doubling time: A fresh look. *Pediatrics, 57,* 469–473.

Nisbett, R. E., & Gurwitz, S. B. (1970). Weight, sex, and the eating behavior of human newborns. *Journal of Comparative & Physiological Psychology, 73,* 245–253.

Piscano, J. C., Lichter, H., Ritter, J., & Siegal, A. P. (1978). An attempt at prevention of obesity in infancy. *Pediatrics, 61,* 360–364.

Report of the National Institutes of Health Consensus Panel on Obesity. (1985). DHEW

Rolland–Cachera, M. F., Deheeger, M., Bellisle, F., Sempe, M., Guilloud–Bataille, M. & Patois, E. (1984). Adiposity rebound in children: A simple indicator for predicting obesity. *American Journal of Clinical Nutrition, 39,* 129–135.

Rosenthal, B. S., & Marx, R. D. (1978). Differences in eating patterns of successful and unsuccessful dieters, untreated overweight and normal weight individuals. *Addictive Behavior, 3,* 129–134.

Shapiro, L. R, Crawford, P. B., Clark, M. J., Pearson, D. L., Raz, J., & Huenemann, R. L. (1984). Obesity prognosis: A longitudinal study of children from the age of 6 months to 9 years. *American Journal of Public Health, 74,* 968–972.

Sveger, T., Lindberg, T., Weibull, B., & Olsson, U. L. (1975). Nutrition, overnutrition, and obesity in the first year of life in Malmo, Sweden. *Acta Paediatrica Scandinavica, 64,* 635–640.

Warner, K. E., & Balagura, S. (1975). Intramural eating patterns of obese and non-obese humans. *Journal of Comparative Physiology and Psychology, 81,* 778–783.

Weil, W. B. (1977). Current controversies in childhood obesity. *Journal of Pediatrics, 91,* 175–183.

Williams, C. L., Hall, W. G., & Rosenblatt, J. S. (1980). Changing oral cues in suckling of weaning-age rats: Possible contributions to weaning. *Journal of Comparative and Physiological Psychology, 93,* 472–483.

5

Dynorphin Shortages and the Compulsions of Bulimia and Hyperactivity

DAVID L. MARGULES
Department of Psychology
Temple University
Philadelphia, Pennsylvania

Two factors most strongly predispose children toward obesity: SES and gender identity. Lower SES females have the highest rates of obesity in American society (Garn, Bailey and Higgins, 1980; Garn and Ryan, 1981 Garn et al, 1981). In this chapter I connect SES setting with psychological dynamics and hormonal events to account for this fact. One may assume that lower SES children suffer significant losses of parental care and attention. Children respond to such losses much as they respond to bereavement: by exhibiting large increases in care-eliciting behaviors. A sexual dimorphism exists in care-eliciting behavior (Raphael, 1983; Gardner, 1976): girls attempt to elicit care and attention by feeding and other care-giving behaviors often directed toward younger siblings; boys engage in attempts to obtain attention by rough and tumble play. When such attempts fail to elicit the desired care, girls may administer the care to themselves by overeating. This produces warmth from diet-induced thermogenesis, and presumably, sedative and stupefacient effects that reduce frustration, promote passivity and may lead eventually to depression. The psychological changes induced by overeating may be caused, in part, by the ability of overeating to release certain messengers such as serotonin and opioid peptides.

The opioid peptides are the type that occupy epsilon-mu type opioid receptors in the body and in the brain. In this chapter I refer to these opioid peptides as stupefacient opioids. In the body, receptors for the

67

stupefacient opioids act to slow metabolic weight loss (Henry et al., 1985; Margules, 1987). These receptors could contribute substantially to obesity because metabolic rate, the most crucial component for the conservation of energy, accounts for almost three-quarters of the total energy expenditure of human adults. In the brain epsilon-mu opioid receptors could promote passivity, learned helplessness and reductions in attention and perceptiveness. Emotionally bereaved boys of the lower SES attempt to obtain care by more active means, involving exercise-induced thermogenesis, hyperactivity, and attention-getting behaviors that may be negative, but are better than receiving no attention at all. Their rough behaviors fail to elicit the care boys need just as the premature parenting roles of girls fail to restore their missing care. Like many addictive behaviors, however, overeating and hyperactivity provide short-lasting temporary relief. The relief boys obtain from overactive behavior may be due, in part, to the capacity of these activities to release opioid messengers different from those released by overeating.

In this chapter I refer to the opioid messengers associated with overactivity as actifacient opioids. Moreover, these actifacient opioid messengers may occupy a different class of opioid receptors than those used by the stupefacient opioids. These actifacient opioid receptors may be located primarily in the brain (delta receptors) (Margules, 1987). For example in the globus pallidus, enkephalin may act as a goad for the resumption of urgent movements that have been halted by dynorphin. During the brief halt, the movement could benefit from sensory feedback, perfected, made accurate and brought under voluntary control (Margules, in press). Without dynorphin movements have an irresistable and compulsive quality such as in Gilles de la Tourette's syndrome (Haber et al., 1986). Shortages of dynorphin may contribute to compulsive hyperactivity, compulsive eating as in bulimia, compulsive drinking as in diabetes insipidus and obsessive thinking when the shortage occurs in the cerebral cortex.

I. Overfeeding Releases Opioids that Promote Hibernation

Although it is well known that overeating induces a stuporous condition in the infant associated with diminished feelings, lethargy and a tendency to fall asleep, no hormonal basis for these sedative and stupefacient effects has been substantiated. In this chapter I consider a hypothesis for a new etiology of obesity in lower SES females. Evidence from experiments in animals and infants indicates that overeating causes the release of powerful messengers such as serotonin and beta endorphin in both the blood and brain. Serotonin contributes to our daily sleep rhythm, a relatively short-lasting state of energy conservation. Opioids of the stupefacient type promote longer-lasting physiological changes in the body and in the brain that are adaptive to famine (Margules, 1979) and serve to move the organism into a prolonged state of energy conservation that resembles hibernation or winter sleep (Margules et al, 1979; Kramarova et al., 1983; Beckman and Llados-Eckman, 1985). Moreover, nalaxone, an opioid receptor blocker, arouses hibernating but not hypothermic animals from their stupefied state prematurely (Margules, et al., 1979, Beckman and Llados-Eckman, 1985). Although humans do not hibernate, they may be influenced by hormones associated with hibernation and have micro-hibernatory reactions in many organ systems including the brain. Two examples of such changes in the body include constipation and respiratory depression. Opioid messengers also prepare the brain for hibernation by establishing a psychological state of passivity known as the learned helplessness condition (Whitehouse et al., 1985). This evidence suggests that the stupefacient effects of overfeeding may be due to the release of opioid messengers which act to conserve energy, promote further overeating and build up the adipose tissue in anticipation of famine. Other neurotransmitters may also contribute, such as serotonin (Yogman et al., 1983), which induces sleep in newborn infants. The release of such messengers in infants could have immediate benefits. Passive, sleepy infants are less demanding, less obstreperous and easier to care for. Lower SES mothers often are overburdened with child care and economic responsibilities for many years. These mothers may find the stupefacient effects of overfeeding tempting to help reduce the effortful job of caring for their children.

II. Overactivity Releases Opioids that Promote Migration

Lower SES families may promote leaness in boys by encouraging physical activities and sports. Boys who have exercised to the point of exhaustion return home ready to rest and fall asleep. Overactivity involves locomotion toward a distant goal usually in a straight line rather than the circular or stereotyped locomotions seen when animals are confined, as in the zoo. Navigation and memory ensure that the individual will be able to return home.

Migration is an exaggerated form of this phenomenon, much the way that hibernation is a prototype for passivity. We do not have much information on the hormonal basis of migration. Migration is an alternative to hibernation that requires a rapid and prolonged energy expenditure. It is not compatible with extreme obesity, although prolonged migration often requires a restricted weight gain. Both migration and hibernation are adaptive to the survival of famine. Although humans do not show the dramatic seasonal migrations of other species, they may be influenced by the hormones for migration and have micro-migratory reactions in many organ systems, including the brain. These reactions would promote the psychological and physiological requirements for migration. These include grouping together cooperatively with other members of the species, motivational persistence to reach a distant goal, navigational skills, risk-taking, courage to leave home, etc. New evidence from the animal literature demonstrates that micro-migratory responses require a class of opioid peptides different from those involved in micro-hibernatory responses. A clearer understanding of the hormonal basis of migration in animals may provide useful knowledge for dealing more effectively with the problems of childhood obesity.

III. Famine: A Natural Selector of Genes for Hibernation or Migration

Americans do not regard famine as a likely possibility. Worldwide, however, famine persists and extracts a deadly toll. In the present era famine kills 10–20 million humans (on the average) each year out of a yearly death toll of 60 million. In past eras, famine has been consistently responsible for more than one-third of the total human death toll. This gruesome statistic places famine among the leading causes of natural selection, and suggests that genes must have evolved in humans and other species adaptive to the survival of famine.

No strong evidence for such genes is available in humans, but in rodents, obesity genes have been discovered. The autosomal recessive gene *ob/ob* in the C57Bl/6J mouse is one such gene. The *fa/fa* gene in the Zucker rat is another. The misty *db/db* gene in C57Bl/KsJ mice is a third. All three genes cause extreme obesity among other changes. We have implicated excessive levels of pituitary opioid peptides, particularly immunoreactive beta-endorphin in the obesity of *ob/ob* mice and *fa/fa* rats (Margules et al, 1978). Excessive opioids may be effects rather than causes of obesity (Holaday, 1985). Nevertheless, these opioids must contribute substantially to the maintenance of obesity, if not to its initiation. Other opioid peptides such as dynorphin and leu-enkephalin have also been found in excess in the posterior pituitary of the *ob/ob* mouse (Ferguson-Segall et al, 1982). Moreover, the *ob/ob* mouse is supersensitive to drugs that act at kappa type opioid receptors particularly in regard to compulsive drinking of water. This suggests that the dynorphin neurons are accumulating dynorphin rather than releasing it. This would create a functional dynorphin shortage that could contribute to the compulsion of drinking. Beta-endorphin also occurs in excess in the pituitary of *db/db* mice. This peptide may have a physiological role in the regulation of feeding. Beta-endorphin rises in the plasma of rats during periods of increased food intake, including both spontaneous nocturnal feeding and deprivation-induced daytime feeding. Moreover, an opioid antagonist, naloxone, suppresses feeding only when beta-endorphin plasma levels were elevated (Davis et al, 1983).

Beta-endorphin also rises in the hypothalamus of rats during periods of increased food intake induced by a palatable meal (Dum et al, 1983). These biochemical results could explain why the opioid antagonist naltrexone suppresses feeding of a highly palatable food much more than that of a nonpalatable food (Apfelbaum et al, 1981). One explanation postulates the existence of opioid receptors concerned with the palatability of food (Cooper et al, 1985; Apfelbaum et al, 1981). Blockade of effects of the endogenous opioid peptides that are released by the ingestion of palatable food could reduce the palatable sensations of foods, particularly sweets. The rats would eat less under the influence of the opioid antagonist because the food did not taste as sweet.

Alternatively, palatability may enhance the potency of opioid antagonists by the promotion of overeating. According to this idea, excessive satiety signals associated with large meals could promote the release of beta-endorphin. This messenger would act primarily to conserve energy by means of reduced energy expenditures in many organ systems, including reduction in respiration, reductions in propulsive peristalsis and lowered body temperature. I have provided a comprehensive outline of the many organ changes that opioids promote in the direction of energy conservation (Margules, 1979) and ultimately hibernation.

Obesity can be promoted substantially by penning animals or preventing them from running and exercising. In lower SES groups penning-in may occur more often in girls than in boys. This would contribute to the higher incidence of obesity in girls. In addition, the stupefacient effects of television need to be considered (Dietz, 1985). Here again the problems and demands of child care are made less effortful by the use of such an approach, and parents are tempted to allow television to serve as a babysitter for many hours each day. If opioid peptides are being released by excessive television viewing, this would explain the stuporous condition children enter into while watching it. Penning-in, of course, effectively prevents children from developing active life-styles.

IV. Migration-like Running May Involve Brain Delta Opioid Receptors

Migrating animals run forward, with few pauses, in a relatively straight line, rather than in circles. They are relatively oblivious to barriers and other external stimuli. The running persists for long periods of time (hours and days) with few pauses. This type of running can be studied in revolving wheels or on a fixed race track apparatus. We are the first to induce this type of running with opioid peptides (Calcagnetti et al., 1987). We accomplished this in obese mice, C57Bl/6J *ob/ob*, an animal with a strong aversion to any type of running, let alone migration-like running. Six-week-old male obese mice have a spontaneous baseline of running of only 45 revolutions per hour. In contrast, lean littermate controls run well over 500 revolutions per hour.

Systemic administration of potent−enkephalin analogues (FK−33824 or FW−34569), substances that act at both mu and delta receptors, produced a dose related increase in running. The obese mice ran forward continuously, oblivious to barriers and other stimuli. Their running persisted for periods as long as eighteen hours. They ran at rates of 250 revolutions per hour. Their lean littermate controls showed no such running even at high doses of FK−33824. Migration-like running of these obese mice could be blocked completely by systemic administration of the following opioid antagonists, all of which have the capacity to enter the brain: naloxone, naltrexone, or MR 2266. In contrast, naltrexone methylbromide, an opioid antagonist given at doses that do not penetrate from the blood into the brain of mice, failed to block FK−33824 induced running.

The data suggest that opioid receptors in the brain are responsible for the FK−33824−induced migration like running in the obese mice. If these effects are produced at delta type opioid receptors, they can be blocked by intraventricular injections of ICI 171,864. If mu receptors are involved, they can be blocked selectively with intraventricular injections of SR58002. Thus, the role of central mu and central delta receptors in migration like running could be assessed. Also, by administering these agents systematically, our idea could be confirmed that peripheral opioid receptors are not involved in this behavior. We have already confirmed the central opioid running hypothesis by means of another technique. Intraventricular injections of doses of FK−33824 as low as 1 nanogram, produced directed running in both obese and lean mice.

V. Future Research Directions

These experiments raise many questions for future investigation. Where in the brain are the opioid receptors for migration like running? Could they be associated with the substantia nigra dopamine system? Are mainly mu, mainly delta, or both receptor types participating? What type of opioid receptor subtype is involved? What prevents the lean mice from showing the migration-like running when the FK−33824 is administered peripherally?

We also have questions concerned with the role of dopamine in this phenomenon. Dopamine occurs in excess in the pituitary of the *ob/ob* mouse (Lorden and Oltmans, 1977). Dopamine metabolism in the nucleus accumbens increases in direct relation to running speed and direction of movement (Freed and Yamamoto, 1985). Moreover, systemic administration of pimozide, a blocker of both the dopamine Type 1 and the Type 2 receptor, blocks the migration-like running induced by intraventricular injections of FK−33824 (Calcagnetti et al., 1987). We would like to know if this is due to the blockade of primarily the Type 1 or the Type 2 dopamine receptor. We could use selective dopamine 1 and dopamine 2 blockers for this purpose. This study has implications for our understanding of the interactions between dopamine and opioid transmitters involved in migration-like running. We expect that future research will provide much information on the pharmacological basis of migration, and this will help to unravel its hormonal basis as well.

VI. Summary

Lower SES girls adopt to parental loss and neglect by overeating and depression which lead to obesity. In contrast lower SES boys respond to such deprivation by becoming hyperactive, which keeps them lean. In each sex, repetitions of the adaptive behaviors lead to the development of compulsions that are addictive and maladaptive. Several lines of evidence clarify how the brain forms and shapes normally free, non-compulsive behavior. A set of dopamine neurons for the initiation of behavior (the nigro-striatal system) is halted temporarily by dynorphin neurons (the striatal-pallidal system). The halt makes time available for choice, sensory guidance and other cognitive functions such as verbalization. Once these events have occurred a set of enkephalin neurons (another striatal-pallidal set) acts to cause a resumption of the behavioral initiative and to reward the resumed behavior. This provides a delayed kind of gratification and a sense of freedom of choice. A shortage of dynorphin activity would abolish the halt allowing the behavioral initiative to rush through to the enkephalin outflow of the motor system in an impulsive and irresistable manner. Similarly an unrestrained serotonin system could cause irresistable deactivations of behavior leading to depression. Finally the beta-endorphin system of diencephalon could cause bulimia if the dynorphin is unable to exert its normal halting action. Apparently the proper development of dynorphinergic opposition to the other opioid peptides depends on "good enough" parental care and emotional training received by children in secure and stable families that model restraint of their own impulses and help their children promote cognitive processing, delay of gratification, and other signs of adult behavior.

References

Apfelbaum, M. & Mandenoff, A. (1981) Naltrexone suppresses hyperphagia induced in the rat by a highly palatable diet. *Pharm. Biochem. and Behavior, 15*, 89−91.

Beckman, A. L. & Llados-Eckman, C. (1985) Antagonism of brain opioid peptide action reduces hibernation bout duration. *Brain Research, 328*, 201−205.

Calcagnetti, D. J., Flynn, J. J. & Margules, D. L. (1987) Opioid-induced linear running in obese (ob/ob) and lean mice. *Pharm Biochem and Behavior, 26*, 743−747.

Cooper, S. J., Barber, D. J., Barbour-McMullen, J. (1985) Selective attenuation of sweetened milk consumption by opiate receptor antagonists in male and female rats of the Roman Strain. *Neuropeptides, 5*, 349−352.

Davis, J. M., Lowy, M. T., Yim, G. D. W., Lamb, D. R. & Malvern, P. V. (1983) Relationship between plasma concentrations of immunoreactive beta-endorphin and food intake in rats. *Peptides, 4*, 79−83.

Dietz, W. H. Jr., & Gortmaker, S. L. (1985) Do we fatten our children at the television set? Obesity and television viewing in children and adolescents. *Pediatrics, 75*, 807−812.

Dum, J., Gramsch, C. H. & Herz, A. (1983) Activation of hypothalamic beta-endorphin pools by reward induced by highly palatable food. *Pharm. Biochem and Behavior, 18*, 443−467.

Ferguson-Segall, M., Flynn, J. J., Walker, J. & Margules, D. L. (1982) Increased immunoreactive dynorphin and leu-enkephalin in posterior pituitary of obese mice (*ob/ob*) and supersensitivity to drugs that act at kappa receptors. *Life Sciences, 31*, 2233−2238.

Freed, C. R. & Yamamoto, R. K. (1983) Regional brain dopamine metabolism: A marker for the speed, direction and posture of moving animals. *Science, 229*, 62−65.

Gardner, R. A. (1976) Psychotherapy With Children of Divorce. N.Y.: Jason Aronson, Inc.

Garn, S. M., Bailey, S. M. & Higgins, I. T. T. (1980) Effects of socioeconomic status, family line, and living together on fatness and obesity. In: R. M. Lauer & R. B. Shekelle, *Childhood Prevention of Atherosclerosis and Hypertension.* Raven Press; N.Y. pp. 187−204.

Garn, S. M., Hopkins, P. J. & Ryan, A. S. (1981) Differential fatness gain of low income boys and girls. *Amer. Journ. Clin. Nutr., 34*, 1465−1468.

Garn, S. M. & Ryan, A. S. (1981) Replicating the income reversal of fatness. *Ecol. Food Nutr., 10*, 237−239.

Henry, L. J., Walker, J., Margules, D. L. (1985) Opposite effects of opiate agonists on metabolic weight loss in mice. *Neuropeptides, 5*, 327−330.

Holaday, J. W. (1985) *Endogenous Opioids and Their Receptors: Current Concepts.* Kalamazoo, Michigan: The Upjohn Company.

Kramarova, L. J., Kolarova, S. H., Ykhananor, R. Y. & Rozhanets, V. V. (1983) Content of DSIP, enkephalin and ACTH in some tissue of active and hibernating ground squirrels (*Atellus suslicus*). *Comp Biochem. Physiol., 74*, 31−33.

Lorden, J. F. & Oltmans, G. A. (1977) Hypothalamic & pituitary catecholamine levels in genetically obese mice (ob/ob). *Bruen Research, 131*, 162–166.

Margules, D. L. (1987) Opioid receptors: An epsilon set in the body acts to conserve energy until a kappa set in the brain permits energy expenditures: Modern concepts of the eating disorders: Diagnoses, treatment, research. (B. J. Blender, B. F. Chaitin & E. Friedman, Eds.) Spectrum Publishers.

Margules, D. L. (1979) Beta-endorphin and endoloxone: Hormones of the autonomic nervous system for the conservation or expenditure of resources and bodily energy in anticipation of famine or feast. *Neuroscience Behavior Revs., 3*, 158–162.

Margules, D. L., Goldman, B., Finck, A. (1979) Hibernation: An opioid dependent state? *Brain Research Bulletin, 4*, 721–724.

Raphael, B. (1983) The Anatomy of Bereavement. N. Y.: Basic Books, Inc.

Whitehouse, W. A., Blustein, J. E., Walker, J., Bersh, P. J. & Margules, D. L. (1985) Shock controllability and opioid substrates of escape performance and nociception: Differential effects of peripherally and centrally acting naltrexone. *Behavioral Neuroscience, 99*, 717.

Yogman, M. W. & Zeisel, S. H. (1983) Diet and sleep patterns in newborn infants. *New England J. Med, 309*, 1147–1149.

Acknowledgments

I would like to thank Nancy R. Walsh, M. S. S. for her helpful insights into the social and psychological dynamics of loss in lower class children. Thanks also to the National Sciences Foundation for supporting my research efforts between the years of 1979 to 1986. I would like to thank my associates, Dr. James Flynn and Joseph Walker, for their hard work, good ideas and for their support of my efforts. Thanks also go to my students, Dan Calcagnetti and Mark Ferguson-Segall for their contributions to the research discussed here. Special thanks to Norman A. Krasnegor and Gilman D. Grave for their interest in my work. This chapter would not have been written without their initiative and encouragement.

6

OBESITY AND FOOD PREFERENCE: MEASUREMENTS IN SEARCH OF MEANINGS

PAUL ROZIN
Department of Psychology
University of Pennsylvania
Philadelphia, Pennsylvania

I. Introduction

The question at hand is whether there is a relationship between food preferences and obesity or overweight (which we will treat together, using the term obesity, even though these terms do not have identical referents). The question can be rephrased: Is there a relationship between how much is eaten and what kinds of foods are eaten? But these two questions are, unfortunately, very different, as the amount eaten is only weakly related to obesity (e.g., Braitman, Adlin and Stanton, 1985; see chapter by Klesges and Hanson in this volume), and actual foods consumed are only modestly predictable from preferences (e.g., Meiselman, Van Horne, Hasenzahl and Wehrly, 1972; Smutz, Jacobs, Waterman and Caldwell, 1974).

Weight, height and skinfold thickness are surely among the simplest and most reliable of dependent variables in the behavioral sciences. Unfortunately, the ease with which one can compute a body mass index leads one to think that this end point represents a unitary phenomenon. Also, because it is a nice hard measure, it is natural to think that it also has a nice physiological underpinning. As it turns out, the various measures of obesity seem to conceal a multitude of etiologies, in which socio-cultural factors play a strong role (e.g. Stunkard, 1975). Furthermore, it is possible that, for cases of moderate obesity, dieting (restraint) is more harmful to health than the maintainenance of above average weight (Herman and Polivy, 1980). And, finally there is now some controversy about the health risks of moderate obesity; some studies suggest that they have been exaggerated (Andres, 1980). The psychosocial costs of obesity (e.g., feeling unattractive, at a competitive disadvantage) may be more significant than the risks to physical health. I raise these troubling aspects of obesity, controversial and familiar to all in the field, because they also plague the study of food preference.

II. Obesity and Food Intake: Preference and Food Choice, Some Parallels

It is also easy to measure food preference. Just ask someone whether they prefer X to Y, or offer them a choice between X and Y, or watch them in the "field" in a situation where they make choices (e.g. a smorgasbord). But this ease is deceiving. Preference is highly contextualized: sweetness preference is a function of the medium (water, juice, etc.), as Pangborn (e.g. 1980) and others have shown us many times. Cultural rules about acceptable combinations are critical: ketchup is preferred with steak, not with ice-cream. (For this reason, questionnaires may be more valid than laboratory measurements of preference, since people usually generate the proper context for questionnaire items.) So, in both obesity and preference, we have a tendency to assume that an easy measurement is a meaningful measurement. It is only in the last 15 years or so that direct measurements of food preference have been contextualized, so that we have begun to move out of the "sugar-water measure" of sweetness preference.

As with obesity, the implication of health as a powerful consequence of food preference is questionable. The major maladaptive consequence of the range of food preferences we see in American culture may be its effect on the quality of life; as with obesity, we may see more denial of pleasure in the service of health than is merited by the data. And finally, sociocultural variables are of substantial importance in obesity, and absolutely predominant in food preferences. For this reason, animal models have limited utility for understanding obesity in humans, and very little value in food preferences.

The bottom line is that food preferences and obesity are deceivingly simple. They are in fact multidetermined and include strong sociocultural components. Their main influence may be on the quality of life, rather than on mortality.

I will briefly review the state of the art in the understanding of human food preferences, in the hope that this may stimulate discussion and the uncovering of linkages between the two fundamental aspects of human eating: What is eaten and how much is eaten.

III.   The Nature of Human Food Preferences

From the point of view of health, the critical measure is what is eaten (dietary pattern), not preferences. It is unlikely that a craving for fats that is unfulfilled because they are more expensive than carbohydrates will have a major effect on health.

We must make a fundamental distinction among *use*, *preference* and *liking* (Rozin, 1979). *Use* refers to what is actually eaten, and can be inferred from statistical data on ingestion by observation, or by self report in any community or country. *Preference* is a comparative measure, and indicates an inclination to choose one food as opposed to another. The two main determinants of *use*, worldwide, are probably cost and availability. Availability doesn't enter into *preference*, by definition (one can't choose something that is not available), and high cost often leads to unavailability. So *preference* predicts *use* only under a limited set of conditions.

We usually measure liking by asking people to check how much they like a food on a rating scale. Sometimes we ask them to tell us which of two foods they like better. But *liking* and *preference* are not the same. Liking is, under certain unconstrained conditions, equivalent to preference, but those conditions are sometimes not met. Hence, a dieter faced with a choice of ice cream or cottage cheese may prefer (choose) the cottage cheese, but like the ice cream better. It is difficult to keep in mind the distinctions among use, preference and liking, but they are fundamental. In many situations, preference is equivalent to liking, and the two terms are used almost interchangeably in much of the literature (and sometimes in this paper). *Use*, however, departs notably from *preference* or *liking*.

IV.   A Psychological Taxonomy of Potential Edibles

Based on interviews and questionnaires, April Fallon and I (Rozin and Fallon, 1980; Rozin, 1984) have identified three basic motivations for the acceptance or rejection of foods: 1. sensory-affective (liking or disliking the taste, smell or appearance), 2. anticipated consequences (beliefs about the beneficial or harmful consequences of eating a food, including both physiological and social (e.g., prestige effects), and 3. ideational concerns (knowledge of the nature or origin of foods). Thus, within any culture (see Table 1), a potential food can be rejected because of bad sensory qualities (what we call a *distaste*), fear of bad consequences (*danger*) or because we know that it is not edible (an ideational rejection, *inappropriate*, e.g., paper or sand). Some foods are rejected for a combination of these reasons. A combination of particular interest is rejection based on ideational factors which also includes a strong negative sensory-affective component. This defines a set of offensive foods (*disgust*, e.g., insects, in our culture).

Potential foods that are ingested usually fall into one of two categories: Positive sensory affective properties (*good tastes*) and positive anticipated consequences (*beneficial*), or some combination of these (see Table 1). Ideational factors are less frequently involved in acceptance than in rejection.

The understanding of the status of a food within this taxonomy, for a given person, may have clinical implications. For example, aversion therapies based on the induction of nausea operate to change a good taste into a bad taste (Pelchat and Rozin, 1982). Such a treatment might be appropriate for an alcoholic for whom the good taste of alcohol is a motive for consumption. However, if the appropriate alcoholic beverage is already distasteful and is accepted primarily as a beneficial substance (e.g., for its effects), aversion therapy would be contraindicated.

V. Mechanisms for the Acquisition of Food Preferences

Humans are omnivorous. A consequence of omnivory is that there are few genetically determined preferences. As far as we know, there are innate tendencies to avoid bitter substances, and probably very strong tastes or oro-nasal irritation. There is good evidence for an innate tendency to prefer sweets (reviewed in Cowart, 1981). There are no other well-documented innate preferences. Thus, we can consider bitter foods as innate distastes, and sweet foods as innate good tastes. In general, infants seem inclined to put just about anything they can into their mouths (Rozin, Hammer, Oster, Horowitz and Marmara, 1986). Thus, much of the acquisition of food preferences early in life, is learning not to eat things like paper, hair, feces, etc.

What causes a substance to become distasteful rather than dangerous? We know of one critical mechanism that produces distastes. If nausea follows ingestion of a food, the food tends to become distasteful (Pelchat and Rozin, 1982). Other negative consequences tend to result in the food becoming dangerous, but not distasteful (Pelchat and Rozin, 1982). If a

Table I

Psychological categories of acceptance and rejection (from Fallon & Rozin, 1983)

Dimensions	Rejections				Acceptances			
	Distaste	Danger	Inappropriate	Disgust	Good Taste	Beneficial	Appropriate	Transvalued
Sensory-affective	−			−	+			+
Anticipated Consequences		−				+		
Ideational		?	−	−		?	+	+
Examples	beer, chili, spinach	allergy foods, carcinogens	grass, sand	feces insects	saccharine	medicines	ritual foods	leavings of heroes or deities

person eats pineapple and gets nauseous, he will tend subsequently to dislike the taste of pineapple. On the other hand, if he gets cramps or a headache or respiratory distress after eating pineapple, he will tend to continue to like pineapple, but avoid it as dangerous. There are surely other mechanisms for acquired distaste. Possibilities include pairing a target food with already bad-tasting foods (Pavlovian conditioning), or negative social connotations (e.g., for a food eaten only by infants). Danger rejections probably result from either personal experience with negative effects of specific foods (e.g., allergenic foods) or cultural information transfer: people are told that certain items are harmful.

The *Beneficial−good taste* distinction is more complex. Again, foods become treated as beneficial, in part, because one is told that they are. The mystery is why foods come to taste good. This problem has been studied by only a few groups (see Birch, 1986; Beauchamp and Cowart, 1985; Booth, 1982 and Rozin, 1984 for reviews of the work of most of these groups). I will review briefly mechanisms for acquired liking (*good tastes*) that have been identified. Pairing with rapid satiety, pairing with foods that are already good tastes, and simple exposure all lead to liking under certain conditions (Booth, 1982; Rozin, 1984). Perhaps the most potent factors are social, as revealed most clearly in the work of Birch and her collaborators. The perception that peers or respected elders like a food tends to make a child prefer that food (Birch, Zimmerman and Hind, 1980). These preferences appear to be based on liking; that is, the foods in question probably become *good tastes*. Birch and her collaborators have also shown that rewarding a child for eating a food tends to reduce ultimately liking for that food (Birch, Birch, Marlin and Kramer, 1982). The argument is that the reward indicates that the respected other who dispenses the reward does not value the food for its own sake and hence employs a reward to induce ingestion. If this finding holds up, it has major implications for child-rearing in the food domain. Birch's findings are substantial but may depend in subtle ways on the context in which rewards are delivered, and on the age of the children (see chapter by Epstein in this volume).

The *good taste-beneficial* distinction is of particular importance because preferences generated by sensory affective motivation (*good taste*) are internalized (the foods are preferred for their own sake) and hence are more stable than those generated by anticipated consequences (see discussion of this issue in chapters by Klesges and Hanson and by Epstein in this volume). I suggest that the best way to ensure good nutrition is to raise children who *like* healthy foods, just as the best way to ensure steady exercise is to get to like the exercise. (In psychology, this corresponds to the distinction between intrinsic and extrinsic rewards.)

There are other mechanisms that have been invoked to account for liking for foods, especially for the reversal of innate dislikes (e.g., hot peppers, coffee, tobacco, heavily salted foods) (Rozin, 1984).

VI. Accounting for the Variance in Food Selection

Another approach to understanding food preferences is to assign individual differences to one of three different origins: Genetic, individual experience, or culture. It seems very likely that culture or ethnic group is by far the best predictor of food preferences. There are no direct data on this point, largely because the conclusion seems obvious. (Differences in diet are also best predicted by culture.) There is, however, substantial within-culture (or ethnic group) variance, and we cannot account for most of it. Genetic differences in behavioral factors (e.g., differences in taste sensitivity) account for a very small amount of variation. (Genetic differences in nutritional variables, e.g., lactose intolerance, may indirectly account for preference variance, mediated by individual behavior or culinary systems.) Most twin studies reveal very little genetic determination of individual differences in preferences. According to common sense, family influences should be the major influence on within-culture individual differences. However, the data reveal very weak correlations (usually in the .0 to .3 range) between parents and their children (Birch, 1980; Pliner, 1983; Rozin, Fallon and Mandell, 1984). Neither sex, nor age, nor personality accounts for much of the residual variance. Individual differences in sensory thresholds or the growth of sensation with stimulus intensity have almost no predictive value for preferences. Many individual differences may result from chance, idiosyncratic events, such as, but not limited to, taste aversions.

VII. Linkages between Obesity and Food Preferences

It is difficult to link definitively two incompletely understood and multi-determined phenomena. And, of course, it is possible that there is *no* relation between obesity and food preference. Or, they might covary without a causal link; or food preferences might contribute to obesity; or obesity might influence food preferences. Furthermore, any relation between these two sets of phenomena might be mediated metabolically (e.g., high fat levels influencing food choice) or by behavior (e.g., perceiving oneself as obese might affect one's food choices, as in the case of a dieter). All that can be done here is to point to possibilities.

VIII. Some Reasons for Skepticism

Insofar as people regulate energy intake well (with obese people accounted for in terms of higher "set point"), the particular foods selected should have no effect on obesity. This may be true for some obese people, but is probably not true for all of them.

Recent work (e.g., Stunkard, Foch and Hrubec, 1986) indicates an important role for genetic factors in obesity. Food preferences, on the other hand, show a very small heritable component in most studies (Greene, Desor and Maller, 1975; Rozin and Millman, 1987; but see Krondl, Coleman, Wade and Milner, 1983), and small familial effects (which provide an upper limit on genetic effects). This disparity argues against a common origin for preferences and obesity.

IX. Some Indications of Relations between Obesity and Food Preferences

It seems unlikely that none of the multiple types of human obesity is related to food preference. In Sclafani's (1984) review of 50 animal models of obesity, three involve food selection (overeating in the "cafeteria−supermarket," or overeating of high sugar or high fat diets). Spitzer and Rodin (1981),in their extensive review of eating patterns in overweight people, identify palatability as the most robust determinant of amount eaten (in single meals) in all people. They also point to a consistent set of data indicating that palatability produces a larger effect on intake in overweight people (related to the externality hypothesis). This is consistent with data suggesting greater importance for flavor and hedonic factors in reactions to foods by overweight as opposed to normal weight persons (Schiffman, Musante and Conger, 1979; Drewnowski et al., 1985). On the other hand, a variety of careful studies of preferences, particularly for sweets, early in life or in adults, by Grinker (1978), Rodin (1977) and others, does not reveal a consistent set of results. Recent advances in preference measurement may bring some consistency to this field. The use of real food contexts as opposed to sugar water, the realization that fats may be more important than sugar as preference determinants, and the realization that relations among flavors and textures may be critical, promise to reduce some variance. Thus, in a recent study, Drewnowski and Greenwood (1983) report notable differences in hedonic ratings of dairy products with different fat-sugar ratios in obese and normal subjects. But we must remember that preference differences surely will account only for some of the obese vs.

normal differences for only some obese people. In order to detect and explore such effects, it would be highly desirable to have a way of preselecting (taxonomizing) obese people into meaningful subcategories.

The basic externality result does not necessarily speak to a difference in food preferences, but to a higher valuation of the perceptual properties of foods as a determinant of intake. In any event, almost all of the studies in the literature use a meal as the basis for judgments. The critical question is the extent to which highly palatable diets (a term which has different meaning for different individuals and in different cultures) produce weight gain when available consistently. The effects of eating more of palatable foods in a single meal can be compensated easily by reduced intake in a subsequent period. The animal data (e.g., Sclafani), and anecdotal reports of weight gain on cruises and the like suggest that palatability factors can induce obesity. But there are little solid data on humans. Naturalistic studies, or longer-term laboratory studies of the type done by Van Itallie or Stellar, Stunkard and their collaborators may answer this question.

X. Summary and Recommendations

At the moment, we have many measurements of preferences and body mass, but we really don't know the meaning of these measurements. In my view, we should face squarely the multideterminancy of these phenomena, and the likelihood that food preferences will account for, at best, a small amount of the variance in body mass. We should also recognize that something very hard to measure accurately, the quality of life, is probably the important end point variable in assessing the importance of changing food preferences or body mass, and in determining the priority of such investigations in comparison with other areas of research. The cyclamate ban and the attempts to ban saccharin made no sense because a very small (if any) mortality risk, a "hard" measure, was weighted extraordinarily heavily against a much larger, but vaguer drop in the quality of life. We cannot let quantification rule over common sense.

In an affluent country, the perception that food selection is very important for health leads to great concern about it, the development of food fads, etc. Most critically, the issue of healthiness of foods, eating a balanced diet, etc., become major grounds for conflict in the family, and probably influence the mental health, or at least the happiness of the family unit. In the United States, parental concern with the food habits of their young children is one of the most common problems faced by pediatricians (Bakwin and Bakwin, 1972). The problem here lies more with the parents. The children who eat only milk, peanut butter, cookies and apples are probably going to do fine, and grow out of these self-imposed culinary constraints (not to be confused with nutritional narrowness) in time. But, when these habits become the focus of family conflict induced by worried parents, the potential for damaging effects rises. One cannot help drawing the parallel to obesity; the risk to health is not so great, but the perception of the risk causes anxiety and generally unsuccessful dieting. To me, the great dangers of deviant food selection (usually not nutritionally risky—one can do well nutritionally at McDonalds) and obesity, especially in children, is damage to important social relations.

Hence, studying how societal values arise and can be changed would be basic to the study of both obesity and food preferences. In my view, the best thing we could do for the obesity problem would be to eliminate the competitive disadvantage and unattractiveness associated with obesity. These values are not operative in all cultures. We would also be well served to communicate to American women the fact that the female beauty ideal of men in their own culture leans more toward heaviness than these women think it does (Fallon and Rozin, 1985). I believe that the best thing we could do to optimize food preferences is to study how societal values (and the culinary traditions of a society) are internalized in children, and to find better ways of educating our population about nutrition.

Another critical area is education. One might start with the introduction of risk-benefit analysis in high school curricula; this is a powerfully important tool for making sane judgments in our complex society. It is surely more useful than factoring polynomials. I think that we can't make too much progress in a society in which many seem to think that it is possible to have completely safe foods or that small amounts of sugar are toxic. I fear that many of the problems we face in food selection, from a public health or fundamental science standpoint, take us into the murky social sciences, and away from the nice control of the animal laboratory.

References

Andres, R. (1980). Influence of obesity on longevity in the aged. In *Aging, Cancer and Cell Membranes, Vol. III, Advances in Cancer Biology Series*. New York: Stratton, Intercontinental Medica.

Bakwin, H., & Bakwin, R. M. (1972). *Behavior disorders in Children* Philadelphia: W. B. Saunders

Beauchamp, G. K., & Cowart, B. J. (1985). Congenital and experiential factors in the development of human flavor preferences. *Appetite, 6*, 357–372.

Birch, L. L. (1980). The relationship between children's food preferences and those of their parents. *Journal of Nutrition Education*, *12*, 14–18.

Birch, L. L. (1986). The acquisition of food acceptance patterns in children. In R. Boakes, D. Popplewell & M. Burton (Eds.),*Eating Habits*, Chichester, England: John Wiley.

Birch, L. L., Birch, D., Marlin, D. W., & Kramer, L. (1982). Effects of instrumental consumption on children's food preference. *Appetite*, *3*, 125–134.

Birch, L. L., Zimmerman, S. L., & Hind, H. (1980). The influence of social-affective context on the formation of children's food preferences. *Child Development*, *51*, 856–861.

Booth, D. A. (1982). Normal control of omnivore intake by taste and smell. In J. Steiner & J. Ganchrow (Eds.), *The Determination of Behavior by Chemical Stimuli. ECRO Symposium* (pp. 233–243). London: Information Retrieval,

Braitman, L. E., Adlin, E. V., & Stanton, J. L. Jr. (1985). Obesity and Caloric Intake: The National Health and Nutrition Examination Survey of 1971–1975 (HANES I). *Journal of Chronic Diseases*, *38*, 727–732.

Cowart, B. J. (1981). Development of taste perception in humans. Sensitivity and preference throughout the life span. *Psychological Bulletin*, *90*, 43–73.

Drewnowski, A., & Greenwood, M. R. C. (1983). Cream and sugar: Human preferences for high-fat foods. *Physiology and Behavior*, *30*, 629–633.

Drewnowski, A., Brunzell, J. D., Sande, K., Iverius, P. H., and Greenwood, M. R. C. (1985). Sweet tooth reconsidered: Taste responsiveness in human obesity. *Physiology & Behavior*, *35*, 617–622

Fallon, A. E., & Rozin, P. (1983). The psychological basis of food rejections by humans. *Ecology of Food & Nutrition*, *13*, 15–26.

Fallon, A. E., & Rozin, P. (1985). Sex differences in perceptions of desirable body shape. *Journal of Abnormal Psychology*, *94*, 102–105.

Greene, L. G., Desor, J. A., & Maller, O. (1975). Heredity and experience: Their relative importance in the development of taste preferences in man. *Journal of Comparative & Physiological Psychology*, *89*, 279–284.

Grinker, J. (1978). Obesity and sweet taste. *American Journal of Clinical Nutrition*, *31*, 1078–1087.

Herman, C. P., & Polivy, J. (1980). Restrained eating. In A. J. Stunkard (Ed.), *Obesity* pp. 208–225. Philadelphia: Saunders.

Krondl, M., Coleman, P., Wade, J., & Milner, J. (1983). A twin study examining genetic influence on food selection. *Human Nutrition: Applied Nutrition*, 189–198.

Meiselman, H. L., Van Horne, W., Hasenzahl, B., & Wehrly, T. (1972). *The 1971 Fort Lewis Food Preference Survey*. Technical Report TR 72–43. Natick, Mass.: United States Army, Natick Laboratories.

Pangborn, R. M. (1980). A critical analysis of sensory responses to sweetness. In P. Koivistoinen & L. Hyvonen (Eds.), *Carbohydrate Sweetners in Foods and Nutrition* (pp. 87–110). London: Academic Press.

Pelchat, M. L. & Rozin, P. (1982). The special role of nausea in the acquisition of food dislikes by humans. *Appetite*, *3*, 341–351.

Pliner, P. (1983). Family resemblance in food preferences. *Journal of Nutrition Education*, *15*, 137–140.

Rodin, J. (1977). Implications of responsiveness to sweet taste for obesity. In J. Weiffenbach (Ed.), *Taste and Development: The Genesis of Sweet Preference*. Bethesda, Maryland: DHEW Publ. No. 77–1068.

Rozin, P. (1979). Preference and affect in food selection. In J. H. A. Kroeze (Ed.), *Preference Behavior and Chemoreception* (pp. 289–302). London: Information Retrieval.

Rozin, P. (1984). The acquisition of food habits and preferences. In J. D. Matarazzo, S. M. Weiss, J. A. Herd, N. E. Miller, & S. M. Weiss (Eds.), *Behavioral Health: A Handbook of Health Enhancement and Disease Prevention* (pp.590–607). New York: John Wiley.

Rozin, P., & Fallon, A. E. (1980). The psychological categorization of foods and non-foods A preliminary taxonomy of food rejections. *Appetite, 1,* 193–201.

Rozin, P., Fallon, A. E., & Mandell, R. (1984). Family resemblance in attitudes to food. *Developmental Psychology, 20,* 309–314.

Rozin, P., Hammer, L., Oster, H., Horowitz, T., & Marmara, V. (1986). The child's conception of food: Differentiation of categories of rejected substances in the 16 months to 5–year age range. *Appetite, 7,* 141–151.

Rozin, P., & Millman, L. (1987). Family environment, not heredity, accounts for family resemblances in food preferences and attitudes: A twin study. *Appetite, 8,* 125–134.

Schiffman, S., Musante, G., & Conger, J. (1979). Application of multidimensional scaling to ratings of foods for obese and normal–weight individuals. *Physiology & Behavior, 23,* 1–9

Sclafani, A. (1984). Animal models of obesity: Classification and characterization. *International Journal of Obesity, 8,* 491–508.

Smutz, E. R., Jacobs, H. L., Waterman, D., & Caldwell, M. (1974). *Small Sample Studies of Food Habits: I. The Relationship Between Food Preference and Food Choice in Navy Enlisted Personnel at the Naval Construction Battalion Center, Davisville, Rhode Island.* Technical Report 75–52. Natick, Mass: United States Army Natick Laboratories.

Spitzer, L., & Rodin, J. (1981). Human eating behavior: A critical review of studies on normal weight and overweight individuals. *Appetite, 2,* 293–329.

Stunkard, A. J. (1975). From explanation to action in psychosomatic medicine: The case of obesity. *Psychosomatic Medicine, 37,* 195–236.

Stunkard, A. J., Foch, T. L., & Hrubec, Z. (1986). A twin study of human obesity. *Journal of the American Medical Association, 256,* 51–54.

7

Determining the Environmental Causes and Correlates of Childhood Obesity: Methodological Issues and Future Research Directions

ROBERT C. KLESGES and CINDY L. HANSON
Center for Applied Psychology Research
Memphis State University
Memphis, Tennessee

Obesity is a serious health problem in the United States because of its high prevalence (Bray, 1976) and relationship to other physical health disorders, including a higher-than-average risk of coronary heart disease (Van Itallie, 1979). Complications related to obesity have a direct relationship to the severity of the obesity (Stunkard and Stellar, 1984). Bray (1976) reported that obesity decreases longevity due to increases in mortality from other conditions such as hypertension, diabetes, arthritis, and operative risk (Drenick, Bale, Seltzer, and Johnson, 1980). Although the specific mechanisms that link obesity and these health problems are not completely understood, many of these complications may be minimized by weight reduction (Van Itallie, 1979; Stunkard, 1984). For example, favorable changes in serum lipid levels may result from weight loss, depending upon pre-treatment levels and amount of weight lost (Brownell and Stunkard, 1981).

The social and psychological consequences of obesity have been well documented (Coates and Thoresen, 1980). There appears to be enormous social and psychological pressure to be thin, and society holds a strong bias against the overweight individual (Allon, 1979; Klesges, Mizes and

Klesges, 1987). Additional stress is placed on people who are obese because they are often held personally responsible for their condition (Brownell, 1982). The obese person may be stereotyped as lazy and lacking in self-discipline (Jarvie, Lahey, Graziano, and Framer, 1983), resulting in a stigma that limits the educational and occupational growth of these individuals (Canning and Mayer, 1966; Benson, Severs, Tatgenhorst, and Loddengard, 1980). These negative stereotypes have been found in children as young as six years (Staffierri, 1967).

These problems are further exacerbated by the fact that obesity often starts in childhood and tracks (persists). Fisch et al. (1975) in a study of 1,786 children, found that 78% of the obese children studied at age 4 were still obese at age 7. Charney et al. (1976) assessed the heights and weights of 366 adults between the ages of 20 and 30 and compared them to pediatric records. They found that the best predictor of adult obesity was weight attained during the first six months. Thirty-six percent of those exceeding the 90th percentile at six months of age were overweight as adults, compared to 14% of the average-weight infants.

Behavioral treatments of childhood obesity have made significant strides in recent years. Epstein, Wing, and colleagues have conducted a series of systematic studies that have sought to increase the treatment effectiveness of childhood obesity programs (e.g., Epstein, Wing, Koeske, and Valoski, 1986). While the results of these evaluations have been impressive, weight loss is difficult to produce and may be beyond the resources of a large segment of the obese population (Volkmar, Stunkard, Woolston, and Bailey, 1981).

Clearly, the prevention of obesity in childhood is a highly desirable and logical treatment objective. For example, Quay and Werry stated (1979): "In the end, the best treatment for obesity would seem to lie in its prevention, which implies the need for much better studies of the eating habits and activity patterns of the *becoming* obese child" (p. 159). Additional studies are needed to pinpoint behavioral targets for intervention and to identify psychosocial risk factors so that obesity can be prevented safely, economically, and efficiently in childhood.

However, it is clear that childhood obesity is a highly complex problem, involving genetic, biochemical, physiological and environmental components (Brownell, 1982; Keesey, 1980; Stunkard et al., 1986). There is recent evidence that adoptees in Denmark more closely resembled their biologic parents than their adopted parents (Stunkard, et al., 1986). However, these findings make the search for determining the environmental causes and correlates of obesity *more* important than before. As indicated by Stunkard et al. (1986): "These findings do not mean that fatness, including obesity, is determined at conception and that ... the environment has no effect. The demonstration of a genetic influence tells us little about possible correlations and interactions between heredity and the environment. We do not know, for example, how a genetic predisposition to fatness may be affected by environmental factors" (p. 196). In any event, for intervention efforts, biochemisty, and genetics are very difficult (if not impossible) to treat, at least on an immediate, individual basis. As a result, we must search to identify *manipulable* risk factors. Unfortunately, the identification of environmental correlates of childhood obesity is both difficult and complex.

Ultimately, the most important research question is: "What causes and maintains obesity in children?" Virtually any *adult* dieter will be able to tell you precisely what causes accelerated weight gain; that is, excessive food intake and/or inactivity. They will also readily inform researchers of the psychological and behavioral consequences of being obese (e.g., social stigma, depression, social pressure to be thin, self-consciousness). In studies of childhood obesity (e.g., Klesges et al., 1983; Klesges et al., 1984; Waxman and Stunkard, 1980), parents will readily and reliably discuss how both they and their children are "different." It has been our experience that few obese people seeking treatment for their obesity view their problem as a solely metabolic or genetic problem. When behavioral changes in dietary intake occur, weight loss reliably occurs in obese individuals (Barnestuble, Klesges, and Terbizan, 1986). Nevertheless, investigators have typically failed to find differences between environmental risk factors (e.g., food intake, physical activity, personality variables such as self-esteem) and obesity (e.g., Huenemann, 1974). As a result of some of these negative findings, some reviews have concluded that food intake and physical activity have little to do with obesity (e.g., Weil, 1977). In this chapter we propose alternative hypotheses to explain the negative and inconsistent findings regarding food intake and physical activity in obese individuals.

The purpose of this chapter is to overview the research on the behavioral and social determinants of childhood obesity. There are three major foci in the present chapter. The first section, *Methodological Issues,* focuses on previous investigations to illustrate issues related to instrumentation, reactivity of measurement in obese subjects, the variability of measures, and limitations of categorizing individuals as "obese" and "nonobese." However, we feel that improvement in instrument and research methodology is only a partial solution to the problem. In the second section, *Integration Issues,* we argue that we need to take a fresh new look at this old problem. That is, we present evidence that obesity (or *obesities*) is a multisystematic problem, involving the child, family, and peer systems. As Hirsch and Leibel (1984) cogently argue, we will probably never find *a* or *the* cause of obesity, because obesity is far too complex to warrant such a simple cause-effect relationship. In the final section, *Recommendations for Research*, we present strategies for studying childhood obesity that focus on increased instrumentation and methodological sophistication as well as take a multidimensional, system approach to this very important problem.

I. Methodological Issues

As will become readily apparent throughout this chapter, there are no easy answers to the question, "What causes obesity in children?" As will be observed, the literature is replete with inconsistent, contradictory, and equivocal findings. No methodological or assessment approach appears to ensure consistent detection of obese-nonobese differences. What we present are *general recommendations* and *research trends*. Exceptions to these trends will also be presented to illustrate the difficulties in studying childhood obesity.

A. Previous Studies have Utilized Insensitive or Too Global Measures

As mentioned earlier, previous studies of environmental determinants of both adult and childhood obesity have failed to find consistent dietary, physical activity, or behavioral differences between overweight and normal-weight children. Unfortunately, a large number of these investigations have used self-report measures that are either previously unvalidated or potentially insensitive to detect subtle overweight-normal weight differences. We would like to discuss this problem by reviewing separately the methodological issues related to obese nonobese differences in (a) Dietary Intake and (b) Physical Activity.

Dietary Intake. The relationship between diet and obesity has long been of interest to nutrition researchers. However, the results of the vast majority of studies of nutrition and obesity fail to find overweight-normal weight differences on measures of dietary intake (e.g., Huenemann, 1974; Berenson et al., 1979), and if differences are found (e.g., Johnson et al., 1956), they appear in a paradoxical direction with obese subjects eating less. For example, in Garrow's (1974) book, the findings of 13 studies relating body weight to food intake were reviewed. Of these, 12 showed the intake of the heavier subjects to be less or equal to that of thinner subjects. These studies, however, have been highly criticized on methodological grounds (Wooley, Wooley, and Dyrenforth, 1979). In several studies, the weight range of the subjects was small. Other studies used questionable self-report measures, small sizes, and laboratory conditions that might be expected to influence normal eating behavior. Despite these methodological problems, as Wooley et al. (1979) state: "the congruence of results is so striking that the burden of proof must be said to rest with those who contend that there is a difference" (p.5).

There have been numerous advances in improving the methodology of collecting dietary information (Beaton et al., 1983, 1978; Frank et al., 1977). Several recent studies (Baecke et al., 1983; Braitman et al., 1985) using this methodology, however, have also failed to find overweight-normal weight differences. An example of the failure to find overweight-normal weight differences in self-reported dietary intake comes from the HANES I survey (Braitman et al., 1985). Directly addressing the problem of poor methodologies and inadequate sample sizes, these investigators analyzed a sample of 6,219 non-pregnant adults whose diets were not restricted or influenced by illness, drugs, or pregnancy. Highly trained interviewers administered a standardized 24-hour dietary recall to all subjects. Diets were cross-checked by a food frequency form for the preceding three months. Results indicated that neither the caloric intake nor the caloric intake adjusted for physical activity levels and age was higher in the obese subjects.

The bulk of the data cited above assessed dietary intake and obesity in adults. The question then becomes, do these negative results hold for children as well? Unfortunately, most data indicate that food intake in children does not reliably relate to obesity status (Weil, 1977). Similar to adult literature, the vast majority of the earlier research (cf. Weil, 1977) can be criticized on methodological grounds. Nonetheless, methodologically sound data from the Bogalusa Heart Study (Frank et al., 1982) indicate no relationship between dietary intake and various measures of adiposity in children.

Studies using specific, detailed, and microanalytic assessments of eating behavior, however, have found reliable differences between overweight and normal-weight children in the *manner*, the *method*, and the *way* they eat. In a model study, Waxman and Stunkard (1980) used direct observation to measure food intake in four families. In each family, there was one obese boy and one nonobese brother whose ages were within two years of each other to serve as a control. A nonobese peer served as the control for school lunch comparisons. The obese boys also ate faster than their brothers at dinner and far faster than their nonobese peers at lunch. The mother served her obese son far larger portions than she did his nonobese brother, and more often. In addition, the Waxman and

Stunkard (1980) study was one of the few investigations that reported that the obese children ate *more* than the normal weight children. Several other studies have failed to find that overweight children ate more than normal-weight children (Drabman et al., 1977; Hill and McCutcheon, 1975; Keene et al., 1981; Klesges et al., 1983; Marston et al., 1976). However, the studies *have* found obese nonobese differences in the amount of time spent chewing and eating food.

The literature also provides examples where the use of microanalytic methodology has *failed* to find overweight−normal weight differences in eating style. For example, O'Brien et al. (1982), with a sample of 356 children, failed to find differences between overweight−normal-weight children in a study of cafeteria food selection and food intake. In an intriguing study, Coates, Jeffrey, and Wing (1978) inventoried available foods in the homes of 65 nonclinical families during unannounced visits. There were few relationships between body weight and the quantity and quality of food stored in these families' homes. Klesges et al. (1984) investigated, utilizing nonobtrusive direct observation, the effects of social setting, type of restaurant environment, relative weight, and sex of 539 adults and adolescents. Results indicated that relative weight was not associated with the number of calories consumed overall. However, the subjects consumed more calories in fast-food restaurants when in groups, compared to when subjects ate alone.

To conclude this section, the results of a number of well-conducted, large scale studies utilizing dietary recalls/records consistently *fail* to find overweight-normal weight differences in dietary intake. As discussed later, these findings may be partially due to such considerations as dietary intake variability, episodic overconsumption, failure to assess physical activity levels or systemic variables, and/or utilizing too global "obese" versus "nonobese" categories. When discrete, microanalytic methodologies are utilized, researchers usually, but not always, find overweight-normal weight differences in eating styles, however (Birch et al., 1981; Klesges et al., 1983; Klesges et al., 1984; Klesges et al., 1986; Waxman and Stunkard, 1980). Thus, dietary factors may indeed play a role in pediatric obesity, although the specific mechanisms of this role have still not been identified.

Physical Activity. While several reviews have concluded (Weil, 1977; Wooley et al., 1979), perhaps prematurely, that dietary intake is unrelated to childhood obesity, there appears to be general consensus, at least with children, that the overweight children are more sedentary than their normal-weight counterparts (Myers and Yeung, 1979; Weil, 1977; Wooley et al., 1979). This relationship is less clear with adults (e.g., Braitman et al., 1985); however, there are several measurement and methodological problems in the assessment of adult physical activity on a large-scale basis (Montoye and Taylor, 1984).

In an early study of physical activity and obesity, Bullen et al. (1964) assessed the physical activity of 109 obese and 72 nonobese adolescent girls engaged in sports activities at summer camp. On the basis of approximately 27,000 behavioral observations, the obese group was far less physically active. Waxman and Stunkard (1980) found that obese boys were far less active than the nonobese controls inside the home, slightly less active outside the home, and equally active at school. In a fascinating study, Brownell, Stunkard, and Albaum (1980) made a total of 21,091 observations of persons going up stairs or escalators in three public places where stairs and escalators were adjacent. Sex, race, age, and weight (obese/nonobese) were unobtrusively rated for each subject. Initially, only 1.5% of the obese subjects used the stairs, compared with 6.7% of the nonobese subjects, a highly reliable difference (p < .0001). A sign, with an illustration of a "weak" vs. "strong" heart was then placed at each location that said, "Your heart needs exercise—Here's your chance." This sign produced a highly significant increase in stair use for both obese and nonobese subjects, although nonobese subjects used the stairs at a level of almost twice that of the obese subjects (14.9 vs. 7.8%, p < .0001).

While the bulk of the evidence indicates physical activity differences in overweight versus normal-weight children, two studies, both using pedometers as a measure of physical activity, failed to find obese/nonobese differences (Wilkinson et al., 1977; Stunkard and Pestka, 1962). These failures to find lowered physical activity differences in obese children, however, could be a function of the pedometers used in the study. Pedometers have been strongly criticized (Bullen et al., 1964) as lacking in precision and having a tendency to malfunction. Two studies conducted in our laboratory (Klesges et al., 1984; Klesges et al., 1985) illustrate this problem. In our first study (Klesges et al., 1984) we used behavioral observation and a simultaneous assessment with a motion-activated activity recorder (i.e., the LSI). The results suggest that the heavier children were significantly less active than the lighter ones as assessed from the behavioral observation data, but no relationship was found with the data from the activity counter. Moreover, inter-rater reliability with the behavioral observation was high (mean Kappa coefficient 0.91). In a convergent validity study of physical activity in both adults and children, Klesges et al. (1985) observed 30 children in a free-play situation while simultaneously wearing two motion activity sensors, a LSI Moving Activity

Monitor and a Caltrac Personal Activity Computer. Results of this study indicated very modest relationships between observed physical activity levels and LSI readings ($r = .40$) and Caltrac readings ($r = .35$). The two motion sensors intercorrelated at very modest levels ($r = .42$). More importantly, relative weight did not correlate to either Caltrac or LSI readings. However, behaviors quantified from the behavioral assessment system reliably correlated to relative weight both concurrently and at a six-month prospective follow-up (Klesges et al., 1985).

Thus, the literature appears to observe consistently, with a few notable exceptions, reliable differences in physical activity between obese and nonobese children. Those few studies failing to find obese/nonobese differences may have utilized insensitive measures of physical activity or may have assessed individuals for an inadequate period of time. While there is general agreement regarding obese/nonobese differences in physical activity, there is less agreement regarding the interpretation of these findings. That is, are lower levels of physical activity in the obese a *cause* or *consequence* of obesity? The answer to this question can only be answered with prospective evaluations of physical activity and obesity.

B.   Obese Children and Their Parents May Be Inaccurate in Their Reports of Dietary Intake and Physical Activity

In a sophisticated study of dietary intake based on 24-hour dietary recalls, Braitman et al. (1985), failed to find obese nonobese dietary differences in a sample of 6219 adults. They offered two possible interpretations for their obtained results. One possible explanation is that obese subjects maintain their greater weight without excessive food intake. The second possibility is that "the estimates of food intake in this study differ in accuracy between obese and nonobese adults, either being underestimated by the former or overestimated by the latter" (p. 732). These authors indicate that "studies to determine the accuracy of dietary surveys on obese and nonobese adults are needed to resolve this question" (p. 732).

It is widely believed in certain clinical populations (bulimia, anorexia) that self-reported food intake is unreliable, as the behaviors associated with the condition are "private." Other health promotion programs such as smoking cessation have great difficulty getting their research published without either biochemical verification of improvement or collateral reports of behavioral improvement (Glasgow and Klesges, 1985). However, it is also widely assumed that obese people readily report their sedentary life-styles and their excessive food intake. Perhaps it is not surprising that researchers do not find differences between obese and nonobese subjects on food intake and physical activity measures!

Anecdotal reports of dietary reactivity in obese individuals are common (Klesges, 1984). For example, in our research on parent-child interactions in the home environment (Klesges et al., 1983; Klesges et al., 1984; Klesges et al., 1986) parents, (and occasionally children) will comment that they are eating the "best meal (i.e., most nutritious) we've had in weeks." In an unpublished masters thesis (Fritsche, 1985), a three-year-old girl's dietary intake *and* weight went down during a *baseline* assessment. In our validational work on motion sensors (Klesges et al., 1985), one morbidly obese adult incorrectly concluded that we were assessing physical activity and obesity. He proceeded to engage in considerable aerobic activity, and, judging from his fatigue at the end of the experiment, he had expended far more physical activity than normal. Clearly, these subjects were reacting to our monitoring of food intake and physical activity and made active attempts at modifying their dietary/ exercise patterns.

Despite the obvious importance of conducting such research on the accuracy of dietary and activity data in the obese versus nonobese, few studies have directly assessed the accuracy of dietary intake across weight classifications. To our knowledge, *no* investigation has assessed the accuracy of physical activity data in the obese. One recent investigation (Klesges, et al., 1985) found that subjects overall tended to overestimate time spent in aerobic types of activity and tended to underestimate time spent in sedentary activities. Unfortunately, biases in reporting were not presented by weight classifications.

There are a few investigations that have attempted to assess the accuracy of dietary intake, however. Early research (Beaudoin and Mayer, 1953) concluded that obese women tend to underestimate their food intake unless they are prodded and assisted by a skilled interviewer. Lansky and Brownell (1982) reported three studies that examined the accuracy and usefulness of food records among dieting obese patients. In the first study, errors in quantity and calorie estimates for ten common foods averaged 63.9% for quantity and 53.4% for calories. Both quantity and calorie distortions tended to be overestimates of actual food quantity and calories. The results of the second study indicated that only 53% of entries in daily food records were specified enough to permit objective estimates of the calories consumed. In the third study, blind raters could not predict weight loss based on subjects' self-recorded behavior changes. This latter finding is in contrast to recent findings (Barnestuble, Klesges, and Terbizan, 1986) that found that self-reported changes in food intake accounted for over 23% of the variance in weight loss at the post-test and six-month follow-up period.

Unfortunately, none of the above studies had normal-weight control groups to determine if normal weight subjects' reports were *also* biased.

Reactivity to measurement can be posited as a reason for the lack of obese/nonobese differences *only if* overweight subjects are *more* biased than normal-weight subjects. Recent evidence, however, indicates that overweight subjects are no more biased than normal-weight subjects in estimating the caloric content of foods (O'Neill et al., 1982; Klesges et al., 1985).

Stunkard and Waxman (1981) reviewed six adult and five child studies on the accuracy of dietary intake in obese versus nonobese subjects, and presented empirical data on six children (three normal weight, three overweight). In their own data, they noted a remarkable similarity between actual versus reported dietary intake in both the normal-weight and overweight children. In the review of the eleven previous investigations, the bulk of the evidence indicates that, on average, overweight subjects are no less reliable in reporting their dietary intake than normal-weight subjects.

Unfortunately, as Stunkard and Waxman (1981) indicate, all of the reports reviewed have methodological limitations. For example, obese and nonobese subjects knew in many cases they were being observed (studies were conducted on metabolic wards, subjects were followed by observers, etc.). In others, the method for assessing "actual" dietary intake may have lacked reliability. In addition, the amount of time from actual intake to recall was very short (e.g., ½–1 hour). Our research laboratory (Klesges, Hanson, and Eck, 1986) recently conducted a careful validity study of the 24-hour dietary recall. This study was with 41 two-parent families, 23 with normal-weight children and 18 with overweight children. Children ranged in age from four to nine years. Subjects were brought into a laboratory and were first given a variety of instruments unrelated to diet to disguise the general purpose of the study. After a few hours, subjects were then given directions to a cafeteria for a free lunch. However, the subjects were not aware that both food service personnel and most of the "diners" in the cafeteria were taking nonobtrusive observations of the child's food intake during the meal. The next day, subjects were visited in their homes and were given a dietary recall conforming to the methodological issues as recommended by Frank et al. (1977). Parents' reports of diets were then compared to their actual intake. Participants were then debriefed regarding the true nature of the study. In no case did any parent have any awareness of the true purpose of the study. The results of this study indicated that parents were quite reliable in evaluating their children's dietary intake. Accuracy did not vary as a function of obesity status of the child or the parent. We are currently conducting a study with adults using a similar methodology to determine if the same relationships hold when overweight and normal-weight subjects recall their *own* diet.

Thus, the bulk of the evidence suggests that obese subjects are at least as reliable in recalling dietary information as normal-weight subjects. However, additional work in this area is needed. For example, in our research, overweight subjects varied greatly in their ability to recall accurately what they ate as compared to normal-weight subjects. To our knowledge, there are *no* published reports on the accuracy of physical activity records of the obese and nonobese. Clearly, research in this area would be a high priority.

Reactivity to measurement is an important issue that needs further evaluation because there may be a negative relationship between the potential reactivity of a measure and its reliability. That is, the most reliable methods of measuring food intake and physical activity involve either direct observation or some method of self-report measure (e.g., dietary recall, dietary record). One of the distinct advantages of these approaches is that they are "direct" and "behavior specific." However, the major disadvantage is that they are highly transparent (i.e., the subject knows the amount of food is the variable being investigated) and thus, potentially highly reactive. One alternative has been to collect more subtle, indirect methods of food intake (e.g., food preferences, food inventories, collection of supermarket slips) and physical activity (e.g., preferred activities, access to and number of facilities that promote physical activity). However, these indirect methods generally suffer in terms of reliability, and it is unclear exactly what these variables are actually measuring.

Finally, reactivity to measurement (i.e., subjects underestimating food intake vs. subjects accurately estimating food intake) may help explain some of the tremendous variability in the food intake and physical activity found in studies of preschool children. It is not uncommon for standard deviations to be larger than the means in these investigations (Frank, et al., 1977). An example of the statistical power problem that results is illustrated below. It has been widely suggested that an excess or deficit of approximately 3500 kilocalories is necessary to either gain or lose one pound (Whitney and Hamilton, 1984). While this estimate is probably greatly oversimplified, let us use it for illustrative purposes. If a child gained an extra 10 pounds of adiposity in one year (above and beyond normal growth), this would be considered a dramatic and alarming increase in relative weight. However, according to the above guideline, he/she would need to eat an excess of only 96 kilocalories per day. Ninety-six kilocalories is less than the standard error of most investigations using a single dietary recall. However, this example assumes a daily, consistent energy imbalance. If, as we postulate below, weight changes can occur rapidly, involving wide fluctuations in daily dietary intake, then our ability to predict obesity is greatly enhanced.

C. "Obese" and "Nonobese" Categories May Be Too Global

As has already been mentioned, the bulk of the evidence evaluating dietary intake in obese versus nonobese individuals has largely failed to find higher food consumption in the obese. One of the many possible explanations for these results is that investigators have collapsed across weight categories and conducted analyses on subjects *current* weight status (i.e., overweight versus normal weight). That is, in any sample of obese people, it is conceivable that subjects are either (a) becoming more overweight; (b) maintaining their obesity; or (c) losing weight. One would expect differences between overweight and normal-weight subjects for dietary intake if overweight subjects were becoming more overweight, while overweight subjects who are trying to lose weight might have *lower* intakes than normal-weight subjects.

Since a large percentage of obese subjects report dieting at any point in time (Klesges et al., 1985), these dieters conceivably could be nullifying differences between overweight and normal-weight subjects. In a recent study, Weber, Klesges, and Klesges (in press) assessed dieting status to determine if differences in dietary intake were found between overweight and normal-weight subjects on the basis of whether or not they were chronically dieting. Subjects were 102 adult females and were classified according to their level of dieting status and relative weight. Careful assessment of their dietary intake at lunch and dinner was obtained. Overall, overweight subjects did not differ significantly from normal-weight subjects in caloric intake. However, when the impact of chronic dieting status is taken into account, a very different pattern emerged. Nondieting, overweight subjects ingested significantly *more* kilocalories than non-dieting normal-weight subjects. Furthermore, dieting overweight subjects ingested significantly *fewer* kilocalories than dieting normal-weight subjects. Most importantly, non-dieting overweight subjects reported eating significantly more than dieting overweight subjects. Thus, the results of this recent investigation indicate that food intake of obese subjects is partially a function of their dieting status. That is, if obese subjects reported dieting, they also reported eating much less than normal-weight subjects. If, on the other hand, they did not report they were dieting, they ate significantly more than normal-weight subjects. Future epidemiological studies investigating the relationship between food intake and obesity should simultaneously evaluate dieting status.

D. Diet Variability May Be Greater With Obese Subjects

It has been observed consistently (Frank et al., 1977; Weber et al., 1986) that the range of dietary intake among obese subjects is much greater than that of normal-weight subjects, as indicated by much larger standard deviations of dietary intake in obese groups. One reason for this variability may be the dieting status of the overweight subject, as indicated above. However, it is also clear that obese subjects are often on a "roller coaster" with body weight, with some subjects gaining and losing hundreds and even thousands of pounds in their lifetime (Brownell, 1982). Dietary intake variability may be a characteristic of these subjects as well. Short periods of large, perhaps massive, food intake are followed by longer periods of dietary restriction. Weight gain in obese subjects may *not* be characterized by a subtle, daily, long-term energy imbalance, but a series of "episodic overconsumption" periods where a large and varied amount of food is consumed in a short period of time (e.g., over the Thanksgiving weekend). The failure to compensate for this overconsumption would lead to rather marked weight increases in a relatively short period of time.

At a recent conference sponsored by the National Heart, Lung, and Blood Institute on smoking relapse (Schumaker and Grunberg, 1986), several models of smoking relapse were discussed. One, the "episodic" model, postulates that abstinence is interrupted by sudden, repeated bouts of heavy smoking. Enough of these episodes or "lapses" produces a person who is "relapse prone," which, in turn, eventually leads to a complete resumption of smoking (Schumaker and Grunberg, 1986). A similar pattern has been noted for alcohol relapse (Marlatt and Gordon, 1985). It seems reasonable to postulate that a similar phenomenon may occur for the person who gains weight. That is, a period of dieting is interrupted by an "episode" of overconsumption. Enough episodes of periodic overconsumption will produce rapid weight gain.

Clearly, this is a very different model of weight gain. The traditional model of obesity has emphasized a subtle daily pattern of chronic energy imbalance between normal-weight and overweight subjects. As mentioned throughout this chapter, the results of these investigations have been largely negative, particularly in adults (e.g., Braitman et al., 1985). The implications of this "episodic overconsumption" model are to evaluate the number, duration, and intensity of the bouts of episodic overconsumption or episodic energy imbalance, rather than to assess *daily* dietary intake and physical activity. The person's *response* to this episodic overconsumption (i.e., resumption of normal intake vs. a short-term self-imposed diet) is also important.

Thus, there appears to be enough evidence to recommend that additional research is needed on episodic overconsumption in the obese and nonobese. A combination of careful laboratory studies as well as epidemiologic investigations will have to be conducted.

II. Integration Issues

During the past two decades, there has been a shift in the way that researchers conceptualize the socialization of children (e.g., Bell and Harper,1977; Bronfenbrenner, 1979). The conceptual shift involves the recognition that children's behavior is a function of the interactions between and within "systems," such as the family, peers, school, and the sociocultural context. Moreover, the interactions among these systems is reciprocal, that is, each system affects and is affected by other systems. Although our discussion of the child's "individual" system, as well as other systems, implies a separation between environmental factors and/or systems, this is purely for convenience in writing. For example, the child's ability to control his or her eating behavior is not an isolated individual characteristic, but is shaped and developed by its interaction with the family and other systems.

Although child clinical investigators (e.g., Garbarino and Crouter, 1978; Hanson, Henggeler, Haefele, and Rodick, 1984) and theorists in the area of behavioral medicine (e.g., Engel, 1982; Schwartz, 1982) have increasingly recognized the reciprocal and systemic nature of human behavior, researchers of childhood obesity have, to this point, employed linear and reductionistic conceptual models. Although such models have provided useful and necessary information in determining factors that contribute to childhood obesity, an understanding of how multiple factors interact and mediate each other in the development and maintenance of obesity is less well understood.

In light of the reciprocal and systemic nature of child behavior and the emerging efficacy of systemic interventions (Gurman and Kniskern, 1986), research findings in the area of childhood obesity are overviewed and discussed from an integrative perspective. In this section, our discussion focuses on three psychosocial systems (individual, family, and, social) that may be associated with the onset and maintenance of obesity. Unfortunately, little data on this model have been collected in the obesity literature. However, we will present research examples from other literatures (e.g., diabetes) to exemplify systemic processes that may be operating in childhood obesity.

A. The Individual System

The behaviors that are associated with dietary intake and physical activity have been addressed elsewhere in this chapter. In this section, we focus on some of the additional characteristics of children that may interrelate with obesity status. These factors include the child's developmental level, self-control, and self-esteem.

1. *Developmental level.* The time frame represented by assessment and treatment studies of childhood obesity is a period of tremendous cognitive, maturational, and developmental growth for the child. For example, in our studies of preschool obesity (Klesges et al., 1983, 1984), the family was the primary socializing influence. However, as children grow older, school and peers also become primary socializers. Developmental changes affect not only the socialization of the child, but also the child's overall physical health (Maddux, Roberts, Sledden and Wright, 1986).

Some of our data suggest that certain risk factors for obesity covary with changes in the child's development. For example, in our early research with two- to three-year-old children, we found that certain *parental* prompts to eat and be active correlated with the food intake, physical activity, and relative weights of children (Klesges et al., 1983; Klesges et al., 1984). In our most recent research with children three and four years of age (Klesges et al., 1986), we found that certain *child*-related prompts (e.g., food requests, food refusals) predicted their level of food intake and physical activity. In other recent work with slightly older children (44 to 81 months), Birch et al. (1981) found that parental reinforcement of the children's dietary intake was *negatively* correlated to the children's tricep skinfold thickness. Although these data need to be replicated in a longitudinal cohort, it raises the possibility that during this brief period, the dynamic relationship between parent and child regarding food intake and physical activity is changing. When the child is very young, the relationships look primarily operant in nature; parents who selectively reinforce food intake are likely to have children that eat more. As the child grows older, his or her ability to control what and how much is eaten increases, though parents still have considerable control over the child.

2. *Self-control strategies.* Another potentially important individual characteristic related to childhood obesity is the development of self-control strategies. Whereas some investigators have hypothesized that obese children have less effective self-control strategies than nonobese children, research findings have been inconsistent. Striegel-Moore and Rodin (1986) suggest that differences in the designs of the studies (e.g., hypothetical vs. real rewards) and developmental considerations (e.g., age and gender of child) make comparisons across these studies difficult. The findings suggest, however, that self-control strategies might be a fruitful area to investigate, especially in light of the recent development of interventions that seem to improve the self-control of children (Meyers and Craighead, 1984).

It would also be interesting to investigate the impact of parental self-control strategies on the child since the development of self-control is related to the child's observation of others (Harter, 1983). Researchers have found, for example, that children will mimic an observed model's resistance to temptation; however, certain characteristics of the model and situation influence the degree of the child's imitation. Perhaps obese children with poor self-control strategies are more likely to have parents who have difficulty delaying gratification, particularly with food. As discussed later, parental discipline strategies also relate to the development of self-control in children.

3. *Self-esteem.* There are conflicting reports on differences in self-esteem between obese and nonobese children (Jarvie, Lahey, Graziano, and Framer, 1983; Kaplan and Wadden, 1986; Sallade, 1973; Strauss, Smith, Frame, and Forehand, 1985). These differences may be due, in part, to the method by which certain variables were derived (e.g., obesity status, self-esteem) and the developmental differences among the samples. When examining self-esteem, it is important to consider developmental differences in the children's view of themselves. Young children (e.g., four- to seven-year-olds) do not perceive themselves in terms of overall self-worth (Harter, 1983). Instead, they view themselves as competent or incompetent with respect to specific *behaviors.* Older children, in contrast, differentiate between specific competencies, such as cognitive (e.g., "How smart am I?"), social (e.g., "How many friends do I have?"), and physical skills (e.g., "How fast can I run?"), as well as general self-esteem (Harter and Pike, 1981).

The developmental shift in children's self-esteem has two main implications for studying the self-esteem of obese children. First, the effects of obesity on self-esteem in the young child may be based on his or her other attributes, rather than obesity. If the child is competent in other domains, such as cognitive skills, the child may feel competent. On the other hand, without significant strengths in other areas, the child might have lower self-esteem based on his or her physical appearance, and perhaps, concomitant weaknesses in physical dexterity. In older obese children, we might expect to find significant weaknesses in their sense of physical competency, but feelings of competency in other areas, such as cognitive skills. This pattern might be similar to adult populations where there are generally no differences found in the general characteristics of assertiveness, depression, and self-consciousness among obese and nonobese groups, but differences arise specifically to physical appearance and weight management (Klesges, 1984). Therefore, investigators need to examine the child's self-esteem across specific areas of competency, especially with older children who may have very different perceptions of themselves across various competency areas.

In some of our research with children who have insulin-dependent diabetes, we found that the child's perceived competence buffered the negative effects of stress on the child's physical health (Hanson, Henggeler, and Burghen, 1987). A similar process may also occur with children who are trying to lose or maintain their weight. Under high stress, children with low self-esteem may engage in poor dietary and activity habits, but stress may not adversely affect those children who have high self-esteem.

In summary, researchers need to consider the developmental level of the child and developmental transitions that may interact with variables associated with the development of obesity. Second, when conceptualizing the role of individual factors in the development and/or maintenance of obesity, it is essential to understand how these characteristics interrelate with other systems (e.g., family relations, stress) that influence the child. Third, the interrelations among these systems are reciprocal, as illustrated by some of the examples cited.

B. Family

The family is a system that is composed of several components (e.g., parental characteristics, marital relations, parent-child interactions, sibling relationships). We address three important areas within the family subsystems: parental childrearing techniques, parent-child interactions related to food and physical activity, and family functioning.

1. *Childrearing strategies.* The impact of parental childrearing styles on child behavior has been examined extensively in both developmental and child clinical research (Maccoby and Martin, 1983). A topic of particular interest is the association between parental childrearing strategies and the development of internalization in the child. Internalization is the process whereby the child develops a sense of internal values which govern his or her behavior. Certain childrearing strategies, such as power-assertive techniques, do not promote the development of internalization in the child and the ability to resist temptation when authority figures are not present. An example of a power-assertive disciplinary strategy in the obesity literature would be putting a lock on the refrigerator to prevent the child from stealing food. This technique does not teach the child to internalize his or her behavior, but to rely on external sources (e.g., rules, authority figures) to govern his or her behavior. Therefore, the child becomes less able to regulate or control his or her own eating behaviors, which causes the parents to continue using power-assertive techniques to control the child's behavior, and the cycle continues.

The importance of the childs' developing self-control over his or her own eating behaviors is also illustrated by an incident that occurred during the following clinical intervention (Fritsche, 1985). Over a period of two months, the observers had made several home observations of an obese four-year-old child, who we will call Susan, to determine if treatment recommendations were followed and were slated to actual weight loss. Interestingly, on at least two occasions, following a low-calorie dinner, Susan went to the bedroom of her younger brother (who was of normal weight) and took his favorite toy. She instructed her brother that if he wanted the toy back, he needed to "ask mother for a popsicle and say it's for you." The young boy dutifully complied with the request, and the "swap" was made. The parents were never aware of this fraternal black-mail. Susan was compliant regarding her diet when her parents were present, but she had obviously not internalized this behavior change. The problem of "sneaking" food when others are not looking becomes increasingly salient as the child becomes older. It is then that the development of internalization is critical.

Parental childrearing strategies that promote internalization also emphasize the use of reasoning that can be categorized as either person-oriented or position-oriented (Bearison and Cassel, 1975; Maccoby and Martin, 1983; Zahn-Waxler, Radke-Yarrow, and King, 1979). Person-oriented reasoning emphasizes the consequences of the child's behavior on others. For example, a child who stole a birthday cake from a classroom party would be told that stealing causes problems and hurt feelings for the rest of the class because there was no longer a cake to give to the birthday child for the celebration. Position-oriented reasoning stresses the use of rules as an impetus for behavior. For example, it is wrong to steal food because stealing is against the law. It appears that person-oriented, rather than position-oriented, reasoning promotes the development of internalization because person-oriented reasoning increases perspective-taking skills, which are related to moral development (cf., Maccoby and Martin, 1983). In using person-oriented reasoning, it also appears that stressing the consequences of the child's behavior on peers has a much stronger impact on the child's internalizing than enumerating to the child how his or her behavior impacts on parents (Hoffman and Saltzstein, 1967; Maccoby and Martin, 1983; Saltzstein, 1976). The usefulness of reasoning that emphasizes the consequences of the behavior on the child (e.g., quitting the soccer team will make you less physically strong and healthy versus you will let the other children down if you quit) needs further investigation.

We are currently developing methods to evaluate parental childrearing strategies so that several hypotheses can be tested. First, we plan to determine whether specific childrearing strategies relate to the development or maintenance of obesity. For example, do strategies that promote internalization in the children also relate to increased self-control and the absence of obesity? Secondly, we will examine the impact of changes in parental childrearing as a function of the child's age. Perhaps there are developmental changes in parental childrearing strategies that relate to lowered risk for obesity.

2. *Parent-child interactions related to physical activity and food intake.* In a study that evaluated parental influences on children's physical activity levels, Klesges et al. (1983) observed that parental encouragements to be active (e.g., "It's such a nice day, wouldn't you like to go outside and play?") were correlated with the child's observed activity levels, and discouragements to be active (e.g., "Your favorite T.V. program is on right now, wouldn't you like to sit down and watch it?") were negatively related to child activity levels. In a follow-up study, Klesges et al. (1986) investigated parent-child interactions related to food intake, as well as physical activity. Thirty preschool children were observed during mealtime and for an hour during free play. Consistent with previous studies, the children's eating and activity were influenced by the parents' selective positive attention to or punishment of those behaviors. Interestingly, parental encouragements for the child to be active were negatively associated with the relative weight of the mother and the father. Moreover, parental encouragements to be active were negatively correlated with parental encouragements to eat.

Several additional studies have examined the impact of parent-child interactions on the food intake of obese children. Waxman and Stunkard (1980) observed that mothers of obese children served their sons larger portions and more frequent servings than their nonobese brothers. The characteristic response by mothers when queried as to this differential food serving was: "he's bigger so he needs more food" (p. 192). Waxman and Stunkard further noted that each mother characteristically "heaped the plate of her obese son while skimping on servings to his nonobese brother" (p. 192). The impact of parental beliefs, attitudes, and behaviors regarding food intake and physical activity toward the obese or "becoming obese" child needs further investigation.

3. *Family functioning.* Hilde Bruch (1971, 1973) was the forerunner in identifying global characteristics of family members and their relations that related to child obesity. Bruch stressed the importance of the interactions between biological and psychological factors, with particular emphasis on family interaction patterns that interfered with the child gaining control over food intake. She also challenged the notion that

obesity is a homogeneous disorder; rather, she described several factors that could interact in the development of the disorder.

There are a few empirical studies that have investigated the link between family functioning and childhood obesity (Loader, 1985). Some studies seem to suggest that obesity and poor dietary habits are related to social isolation and dependent family relations (Bullen, Monello, Cohen, and Mayer, 1963; Hammar et al., 1972; Kintner, Boss, and Johnson, 1981). For example, Kintner and colleagues found that the mothers' perception of independence was positively related to the nutritional content of the family's diet. The researchers postulate that the family environment is exhibited in the family's dietary habits (e.g., mothers who feel independent engage in healthy dietary habits). These findings may also reflect bidirectional influences, that is, healthy dietary habits may influence the mothers' overall well-being and ability to function independently.

Family conflict also seems to be associated with the physical health of family members. Some of our preliminary findings suggest that mothers and children tend to weigh more in conflictual families (Hanson, Klesges, and Eck, 1986b). In addition, low cohesiveness (e.g., emotional bonding between family members) and low expressiveness (e.g., acting openly and expressing feelings directly) among family members related to high blood pressure/heart rate in parents. Again, these findings may reflect bidirectional influences. For example, parents who have high blood pressure may perceive more stress at their jobs and may spend less time at home, which could contribute to a less cohesive and expressive family environment. In any case, these results further illustrate the contextual nature of a family member's health.

In addition to the role of the family environment, our preliminary data indicate that certain parental characteristics are linked with child obesity (Hanson, Klesges, and Eck, 1986a). For example, maternal depression positively correlated with child weight. Although the child's weight could affect the mother's mood, or a moderating variable could impact upon both the child's weight and mother's mood, it is also quite possible that the mother's mood affects her behaviors, which in turn, impact upon the child and his or her health. For example, mothers who are depressed might not be as physically active or as likely to engage in physical activity with their children. This is just one example of an indirect pathway by which maternal depression could adversely affect the child's health.

Many child behavior problems are closely linked with family relations. As such, Epstein (1986) emphasized the importance of whether the parent and child are seen together or separately during child obesity treatment. Epstein's attention to the role of parents in treatment is important;

however, from a systemic perspective, the key is not the parent's physical presence in treatment, but the therapist's attempts to modify parent-child relations that contribute to the problem.

From a multisystemic therapeutic perspective, it is sometimes better to treat both parents and children together, and other times it is necessary to see the child alone. For example, it is occasionally necessary to intervene with the parent and child separately to encourage the child's independence, as well as to focus on issues central to the parent. During adolescence, the adolescent actively exercises his or her newly developed cognitive capabilities of understanding the possibilities and choices in life. Because of these developmental changes, parents have less control over the adolescent's behavior. A disruption in this normal emancipation process often results in adolescent behavior problems, including those related to weight maintenance (e.g., anorexia nervosa). Therefore, it is not surprising that Brownell, Kelman, and Stunkard (1983) found that separating the parent and adolescent in treatment versus seeing them together related to better short-and long-term weight loss. As the researchers hypothesize, it was most likely the manipulation of the parent-child relationships that led to these differences, not the mere presence or absence of the parent. It is the empirical investigation of the qualitative aspects of family relations that is clearly needed.

In summary, family relations appear linked to family members cardiovascular health (e.g., obesity, blood pressure). Further investigations and replications appear to be of high priority.

C. Peer Relations

Several research studies have examined whether obese children are more often rejected by their peers (for a review, see Jarvie et al., 1983). Physical appearance is an important factor in the development of interpersonal relationships and acceptance from others. Because thinness is highly valued and seen as attractive in our society, obesity may place the child at increased risk for social maladjustment. We now turn our attention to the association between physical attractiveness and peer relations in childhood.

Young children's views of others are largely based on "concrete" categories, such as physical appearance and possessions. Young children are also able to acknowledge differences and preferences for certain physical characteristics. For example, Dion (1973) found that children three to five years of age respond with society's stereotypes regarding facial attractiveness (e.g., "which one is prettier?"). In light of the fact that young children tend to categorize and discriminate between their peers on global physical characteristics, young obese children may be treated differently from their normal-weight counterparts. For example, among preschoolers, prosocial behaviors (e.g., friendliness, nonaggressiveness) are more frequently attributed to attractive versus unattractive children, and negative behaviors are more likely associated with unattractive children (Adams and Crane, 1980; Dion, 1973; Dion and Berscheid, 1974). Moreover, from preschoolers to adolescents, children view an attractive child as a better candidate for a friend than an unattractive child (Cavior and Dokecki, 1973; Dion, 1973; Langlois and Stephan, 1977). Teachers also have different expectations of attractive versus unattractive children, particularly children with whom they are unfamiliar (Hartup, 1983). These studies indicate a substantial advantage for children who are perceived as attractive by significant people in the child's social network.

It is not until children are older that they learn to identify and describe more abstract qualities of the person, such as beliefs and interpersonal characteristics (Flavell, 1977). However, even though adolescents are able to appreciate people's intrapersonal characteristics and the interpersonal qualities in relationships, physical attractiveness is still very important during adolescence. The adolescent becomes more aware of his or her body and physical maturation related to issues of sexuality and dating. Adolescents also become increasingly concerned about being a part of a social group that has similar characteristics and interests. It seems likely that the obese adolescent would experience some peer rejection that is associated with physical attractiveness and/or physical dexterity, such as dating, cheerleading, and certain sports.

In light of these findings, does attractiveness affect the child's acceptance from peers? Clearly, further research is needed to unravel some of the more complicated issues involved. For example, the impact of attractiveness on social interaction becomes more complicated when the children are acquaintances versus stangers, when the gender of the child is taken into account, when the situational context is explored (e.g., is the child being chosen for an athletic team or to go to a movie), when the degree of disfigurement is examined (e.g., the extent of the obesity, facial attractiveness with an obese body), and when the perceived responsibility for the unattractiveness is blamed on the child versus on some physiological disorder which the child has no control over (Hartup, 1983; Jarvie et al., 1983). Overall, the research suggests that it is advantageous to have an attractive face and body, but the extent to which it is disadvantageous to have an unattractive face and an endomorphic physique is less clear (Hartup, 1983; Jarvie et. al., 1983).

Another important area related to peers is the extent to which the peer group supports healthy behaviors. For example, is the peer group physically active or sedentary? Do the peer groups' social activities focus around food? The social setting appears to be an important contributor to food intake (Streigel-Moore and Rodin, 1983). For example, Stunkard and Mazer (1978) found that the frequency of obese adults dining at a restaurant was greatly increased when a smorgasbord was served. The impact of various settings on behaviors in children seems a fruitful area to explore, particularly with the powerful impact of peers within these settings.

D. Summary

We have discussed the importance of examining the multisystemic influences on childhood obesity. Individual, family, and peer characteristics are likely to interact to produce and maintain obesity in the child. However, it is important to note that the factors associated with onset of obesity may be very different than the factors associated with its maintenance. For example, investigators have generally found reduced levels of activity among obese children with cross-sectional research designs. What is unclear is whether reduced levels of physical activity is an etiological risk or merely a consequence of obesity. Does obesity in children cause difficulties in peer relations, or do children who have peer difficulties become obese? Observing children longitudinally will allow us to answer some of these important questions and ultimately to help in the treatment of this difficult and refractory disorder. In addition, we need to consider the multisystemic factors that contribute to the onset and maintenance of the obesity. Neglecting an important system that impacts upon the child could easily sabotage treatment efforts.

III. Recommendations for Future Research

In summary, these methodological and integrative issues are important in understanding results obtained. Possible solutions are difficult, time-consuming, and expensive. Our research recommendations are summarized below:

(1) Encourage and support additional longitudinal research to identify psychosocial correlates of childhood obesity. The acquisition of obesity is a longitudinal phenomenon that probably involves subtle, discrete, and microanalytic food intake, physical activity, and psychosocial changes that result in obesity over a period of time. What are needed are prospective evaluations to predict relative weight, and more importantly, relative

weight change over time. It is important also to note that the factors associated with the *onset* of obesity may be very different from the factors associated with the *maintenance* of obesity. For example, we have mentioned that researchers have generally found reduced levels of physical activity in obese children. What is unclear in these cross-sectional studies is whether a reduced level of physical activity is an etiological risk factor or merely a consequence of obesity.

(2)   Utilize a multi-trait multi-method assessment methodology. Self-report, observational, behavioral, and environmental assessments each have their unique advantages and disadvantages. This methodology will assist in improving reliability, temporal stability, and discriminant validity of the measures. There is ample evidence that multiple assessment/multiple occasion measurements are superior to single behavioral samples.

(3)   Conduct reliability, validity, and generalizability studies prior to finalizing any research protocol. This may assist in striking a balance between the number of behavioral samples per subject and the labor-intensive nature of the project.

(4)   Additional studies of reactivity of measurement in obese and nonobese subjects are needed. There are but few published reports on the accuracy of dietary variables in obese subjects, and, to our knowledge, there are no published reports on the accuracy of physical activity variables.

(5)   Research should begin on the "episodic overconsumption" model of obesity and its possible relationship to the onset and maintenance of weight gain. Available laboratory data (e.g., Polivy, 1980) suggest that this model of obesity is certainly worth pursuing.

(6)   Carefully consult the developmental and clinical literature to evaluate potential influences and moderators of food intake, physical activity, and relative weight. For example, childrearing style may interact with child food preferences in predicting childhood obesity. Child preference of sugary food in conjunction with a permissive and/or ineffective parenting style may predict childhood obesity, whereas neither variable by itself may predict obesity. Predictors of childhood obesity may also be age and/or developmentally related. For example, predictors of childhood obesity at one age (e.g., parental encouragements to eat) may not predict obesity at another age (Klesges et al., 1986).

References

Adams, G. R. & Crane, P. (1980). An assessment of parents' and teachers' expectations of preschool children's social preference for attractive or unattractive children and adults. *Child Development, 51,* 224–231.

Allon, N. (1979). Self-perceptions of the stigma of overweight in relationship to weight-losing patterns. *The American Journal of Clinical Nutrition, 32,* 470–480.

Baecke, J. A. H., van Staveren, W. A., & Burema, J. (1983). Food consumption, habitual physical activity, and body fatness in young Dutch adults. *The American Journal of Clinical Nutrition, 37,* 278–286.

Barnestuble, J. A., Klesges, R. C., & Terbizan, D. (1986). Predictors of weight loss in a behavioral treatment program. *Behavior Therapy, 17,* 288–294.

Bearison, D. J., & Cassel, T. Z. (1975). Cognitive decentration and social codes: Communication effectiveness in young children from differing family contexts. *Developmental Psychology, 11,* 29–36.

Beaton, G. H., Milner, J., Corey, P., McGuire, V., Cousins, M., Stewart, E., deRamos, M., Hewitt, D., Grambsch, P. V., Kassim, N., & Little, J. A. (1978). Sources of variance in 24-hour dietary recall data: Implications for nutrition study design and interpretation. *The American Journal of Clinical Nutrition, 32,* 2546–2559.

Beaton, G. H., Milner, J., McGuire, V., Feather, T. E., & Little J. A. (1983). Sources of variance in 24-hour dietary recall data: Implications for nutrition study design and interpretation. Carbohydrate sources, vitamins, and minerals. *The American Journal of Clinical Nutrition, 37,* 986–995.

Beaudoin, R. & Mayer, J. (1953). Food intakes of obese and non-obese women. *Journal of the American Dietetics Association, 29,* 29–33.

Bell, R. Q., & Harper, L. V. (1977). *Child Effects on Adults.* Hillsdale, NJ: Erlbaum.

Benson, P. L., Severs, D., Tatgenhorst, J., & Loddengaard, N. (1980). The social cost of obesity: A non-reactive field study. *Social Behavior and Personality, 8,* 91–96.

Berenson, G. S., Blonde, C. V., Farris, R. P., Foster, T. A., Frank, G. C., Srinivasan, S. R., Voors, A. W., & Webber, L. S. (1979). Cardiovascular disease risk factor variables during the first year of life. *American Journal of Diseases in Children, 122,* 1049–1057.

Birch, L. L., Marlin, D. W., Kramer, L., & Peyer, C. (1981). Mother-child interaction patterns and the degree of fatness in children. *Journal of Nutrition Education, 13,* 17–21

Braitman, L. E., Adlin, E. V., & Stanton, J. L., Jr. (1985). Obesity and caloric intake: The National Health and Nutrition Examination Survey of 1971–1975 (HANES I). *Journal of Chronic Diseases, 38,* 727–732.

Bray, G. (1976). *The Obese Patient.* Philadelphia: W. B. Saunders Company.

Bronfenbrenner U. (1979). *The Ecology of Human Development.* Cambridge, MA: Harvard University.

Brownell, K. D. (1982). Obesity: Understanding and treating a serious prevalent and refractory disorder. *Journal of Consulting and Clinical Psychology, 50,* 820–840.

Brownell, K. D., Kelman, J. H., & Stunkard, A. J. (1983). Treatment of obese children with and without their mothers: Changes in weight and blood pressure. *Pediatrics, 71,* 515–523.

Brownell, K. D. & Stunkard, A. J. (1981). Differential changes in plasma high density lipoprotein-cholesterol levels in obese men and women during weight reduction. *Archives of Internal Medicine, 141,* 1142–1146.

Brownell, K. D., Stunkard, A. J., & Albaum, J. M. (1980) Evaluation and modification of exercise patterns in the natural environment. *American Journal of Psychiatry, 137,* 1540–1545.

Bruch, H. (1971). Family transactions in eating disorders. *Comprehensive Psychiatry, 12,* 238–248.

Bruch, H. (1973). *Eating Disorders.* NY: Basic Books.

Bullen, B. A., Monello, L. F., Cohen, H., & Mayer, J. (1963). Attitude toward physical activity, food and family in obese and non-obese adolescent girls. *American Journal of Clinical Nutrition, 12,* 1–11.

Bullen, B. A., Reed, R. B., & Mayer, J. (1964). Physical activity of obese and non-obese adolescent girls appraised by motion picture sampling. *American Journal of Clinical Nutrition, 14,* 211–223.

Canning, H. & Mayer, J. (1966). Obesity – Its possible effect on college acceptance. *The New England Journal of Medicine, 275,* 1172–1174.

Cavior, N., & Dokecki, P. R. (1973). Physical attractiveness, perceived attitude similarity, and academic achievement as contributors to interpersonal attraction among adolescents. *Developmental Psychology, 9,* 44–54.

Charney, E., Goodman, H. C., McBride, M., Lyon, B., & Pratt, R., (1976). Childhood antecedents of adult obesity. *New England Journal of Medicine, 295,* 6–9.

Coates, T. J. & Thoresen, C. E. (1980). Obesity in children and adolescents: The problem belongs to everyone. In B. Lahey & A. Kazdin (Eds.), *Advances in Child Clinical Psychology, Vol. 3.* N.Y.: Plenum.

Coates, T. J., Jeffrey, R. W. & Wing, R. R. (1978). The relationship between persons' relative body weights and the quality and quantity of food stored in their homes. *Addictive Behaviors, 3,* 179–184.

Dion, K. K. (1973). Young children's stereotyping of facial attractiveness. *Developmental Psychology, 9,* 183–198.

Dion, K. K., & Berscheid, E. (1974). Physical attractiveness and peer perception among children. *Sociometry, 37,* 1–12.

Drabman, R. S., Cordua, G. D., Hammer, D., Jarvie, G. J., & Horton, W. (1977). Eating styles of obese and non-obese black and white children in a naturalistic setting. *Addictive Behaviors, 2,* 83–86.

Drenick, E. J., Bale, G. S., Seltzer, F., & Johnson, D. G. (1980). Excessive mortality and causes of death in morbidly obese men. *Journal of the American Medical Association, 243,* 443–445.

Engel, G. I. (1982). The biopsychosocial model and medical education, *New England Journal of Medicine, 306,* 802–805.

Epstein, L. H. (1986). Treatment of childhood obesity. In Brownell, K. D., & Foreyt, J. P. (Eds.), *Handbook of Eating Disorders: Physiology, Psychology, and Treatment of Obesity, Anorexia, and Bulimia*(pp. 159–179). NY: Basic Books.

Epstein, L. H., Wing, R. R., Koeske, R., & Valoski, A. (1986). Effect of parent weight on weight loss in obese children. *Journal of Consulting and Clinical Psychology, 54,* 400–401.

Fisch, R. O., Bilek, M. K., & Ulstrom, R. (1975). Obesity and leanness at birth and their relationship to body habitus in early childhood. *Pediatrics, 56,* 521–528.

Flavell, J. H. (1977). *Cognitive Development.* NJ: Prentice-Hall.

Foreyt, J. P., Mitchell, R. E., Garner, D. T., Gee, M., Scott, L. W., & Gotto, A. M. (1982). Behavioral treatment of obesity: Results and limitations. *Behavior Therapy, 13,* 153–161.

Frank, G. C., Webber., L. S., & Webber, G. S. (1982). Dietary studies of infants and children: The Bogalusa Heart Study. In T.J. Coates, A.C. Peterson, & C. Perry (Eds.), *Promoting Adolescent Health: A Dialogue on Research and Practice.* New York: Academic Press.

Frank, G. C., Voors, A. W., Schilling, P. E., & Berenson, G. L. (1977). Dietary studies in rural school children in a cardiovascular survery. *Journal of the American Dietetic Association, 71,* 31–35.

Frank, G. C., Berenson, G. S., Schilling, P. E., & Moore, M. C. (1977). Adapting the 24-hour recall for epidemiologic studies of school children. *Journal of the American Dietetic Association, 71,* 26–31.

Fritsche, B. M. (1985). *Treatment of Childhood Obesity Based on Assessment of Individual Risk Factors.* Unpublished masters thesis, North Dakota State University, Fargo, ND.

Garbarino, J., & Crouter, A. (1978). Defining the community context for parent-child relations: The correlates of maltreatment, *Child Development, 49,* 604–619.

Garrow, J. (1979). *Energy Balance and Obesity in Man.* New York: American Elsevier.

Glasgow, R. E. & Klesges, R. C. (1985). Smoking intervention programs in the workplace. Chapter (12) published in the U.S. Department of Health, Education, and Welfare's: *The Health Consequences of Smoking Cancer and Chronic Lung Disease in the Workplace. A Report of the Surgeon General.* U.S. Department of Health and Human Services, Public Health Service, Office of the Assistant Secretary for Health, Office on Smoking and Health, DHHS Pub. No. (85-50207).

Gurman, A. S., & Kniskern, D. P. (1986). Research on the process and outcome of marital and family therapy. In S. Garfield, & A. Bergin (Eds.), *Handbook of Psychotherapy and Behavior Change* (3rd ed.). NY:Wiley.

Hammar, S. L., Campbell, M. M., Campbell, A., Moores, N. L., Sareen, C., Gareis, F. J., & Lucas, M. P. H. (1972). An interdisciplinary study of obesity. *Journal of Pediatrics, 80,* 373–383.

Hanson, C. L., Henggeler, S. W., & Burghen, G. A. (1987). Social competence and parental support as mediators of the link between stress and metabolic control in adolescents with IDDM. *Journal of Consulting and Clincial Psychology, 55,* 529–533.

Hanson, C. L., Henggeler, S. W., Haefele, W. F., & Rodick, J. D. (1984). Demographic, individual, and family relationship correlates of serious and repeated crime among adolescents and their siblings. *Journal of Consulting and Clinical Psychology, 52,* 528–538.

Hanson, C. L., Klesges, R. C., & Eck, L. H. (1986a). Coping behavior: Effects on cardiovascular functioning. Submitted for publication.

Hanson, C. L., Klesges, R. C., & Eck, L. H., & Cigrang, J. A. (1986b). A link between cardiovascular health and family functioning. Submitted for publication.

Harter, S. (1983). Developmental perspective on the self-system. In P. H. Mussen (Ed.), E. M. Hetherington (vol. Ed), *Handbook of Child Psychology (4th ed.): Socialization, Personality, and Social Development* (Vol. IV pp. 276–385). NY: John Wiley & Sons.

Harter, S., & Pike, R. (1981). *The Pictorial Percieived Competence Scale for Young Children.* Unpublished manuscript, University of Denver.

Hartup, W. W. (1983). Peer relations. In P. H. Mussen (Ed.), E. M. Hetherington (Vol. Ed.), *Handbook of child psychology (4th ed.): Socialization, Personality, and Social Development* (Vol. IV pp. 103–196). NY: John Wiley & Sons.

Hill, S. W. & McCutcheon, B. (1975). Eating response of obese and nonobese humans during dinner meals. *Psychosomatic Medicine, 37,* 395–401.

Hirsch, J. & Leibel, R. L. (1984). What constitutes a sufficient psychobiologic explanation for obesity. In A. Stunkard & E. Stellar (Eds.), *Eating and its Disorders.* New York: Raven.

Hoffman, M. L., & Saltzstein, H. D. (1967). Parent discipline and the child's moral development. *Journal of Personality and Social Psychology, 5,* 45–57.

Huenemann, R. L. (1974). Environmental factors associated with preschool obesity. *Journal of the American Dietetic Association, 64,* 480–487.

Jarvie, G. J., Lahey, B., Graziano, W., & Framer, E. (1983). Childhood obesity and social stigma: What we know and what we don't know. *Developmental Review, 3,* 237–273.

Johnson, M. L., Burke, B. S., & Mayer, J. (1956). Relative importance of inactivity and over-eating in the energy balance of obese high school girls. *American Journal of Clinical Nutrition, 4,* 37–44.

Kaplan, K. M., & Wadden, T. A. (1986). Childhood obesity and self-esteem. *Behavioral Pediatrics, 109,* 367–370.

Keane, T. M., Gellar, S. E., & Schreirer, C. J. (1981). A parametric investigation of eating styles in obese and nonobese children. *Behavior Therapy, 12,* 280–286.

Keesey, R. E. (1980). A set-point analysis of the regulation of body weight. In A. J. Stunkard (Ed.), *Obesity*. Philadelphia: Saunders.

Kintner, M., Boss, P. G., & Johnson, N. (1981). The relationship between dysfunctional family environments and family member food intake. *Journal of Marriage and the Family, 43*, 633–641.

Klesges, R. C. (1984). Obesity and personality: Global versus specific measure? *Behavioral Assessment, 6*, 347–356.

Klesges, R. C., Coates, T. J., Holzer, B., Moldenhauer, L. M., Woolfrey, J., & Vollmer, J. (1983). Parental influences on children's eating behavior. *Journal of Applied Behavior Analysis, 16*, 371–378.

Klesges, R. C , Bartsch, D., Norwood, J. D., Kautzman, D., & Haugrud, S. (1984). The effects of selected social and environmental variables on the eating behavior of adults in the natural environment. *International Journal of Eating Disorders, 3*, 35–41.

Klesges, R. C., Beatty, W. W., & Berry, S. L. (1985). Some behavioral, attitudinal, and perceptual correlates of obesity in a university population. *International Journal of Eating Disorders, 4*, 237–245.

Klesges, R. C., Coates, T. J., Moldenhauer-Klesges, L. M., Holzer, B., Gustavson, J., & Barnes, J. (1984). The FATS: And observational system for assessing physical activity in children and associated parent behavior. *Behavioral Assessment, 6*, 333–345.

Klesges, R. C., Hanson, C. L., & Eck, L. H. (1986). *Caloric intake estimates of overweight versus normal weight children: A nonobtrusive field study.* Manuscript in preparation.

Klesges, R. C., Hanson, C. L., & Eck, L. H. (1986). *The effects of obesity status memory functioning levels on the accuracy of dietary intake.* Manuscript in preparation.

Klesges, R. C., Mizes, J. S. & Klesges, L. M., (1987). Dieting strategies in a college population. *International Journal of Eating Disorders, 6*, 71–79.

Klesges, R. C., Klesges, L. M., Swenson, A. M., & Pheley, A. (1985). A validation of two motion sensors in the prediction of child and adult physical activity levels. *American Journal of Epidemiology, 122*, 400–410.

Klesges, R. C., Klesges, L. M., Weber, J., & Swenson, A. (1986). *Parent-Child Interactions and Eating Behavior.* Unpublished manuscript, North Dakota State University, Fargo, ND.

Klesges, R. C., Malott, J. M., Boschee, P. F., & Weber, J.M. (1986). The effects of parental influences on children's food intake, physical activity, and relative weight. *International Journal of Eating Disorders. 5*, 335–346.

Langlois, J. H., & Stephan, C. (1977). The effects of physical attractiveness and ethnicity on children's behavioral attributions and peer preferences. *Child Development, 48*, 1694–1698.

Lansky, D. & Brownell, K. D. (1982). Estimates of food quantity and calories: Errors in self-report among obese patients. *American Journal of Clinical Nutrition, 35*, 727–732.

Loader, P. J. (1985). Childhood obesity: The family perspective. *International Journal of Eating Disorders, 4*, 211–225.

Maccoby, E. E., & Martin, J. A. (1983). Socialization in the context of the family; parent-child interaction. In Paul H. Mussen (Ed.), E. M. Hetherington (Vol. Ed.), *Handbook of Child Psychology (4th ed.): Socialization, Personality, and Social Development* (Vol. IV pp. 1–101). NY: John Wiley & Sons.

Maddux, J. E., Roberts, M. C., Sledden, E. A., & Wright, L. (1986). Developmental issues in child health psychology. *American Psychologist, 41*, 25–34.

Marlatt, G. A. & Gordon, J. R. (1985). *Relapse Prevention: Maintenance Strategies in the Treatment of Addictive Behaviors.* New York: Guilford.

Marston, A. R., London, P., & Cooper, L. M. (1976). A note on the eating behavior of children varying in weight. *Journal of Child Psychology and Psychiatry, 17*, 221–224.

Meyers, A. W., & Craighead, W. E. (Eds.) (1984). *Cognitive Behavior Therapy with Children*. NY: Plenum.

Montoye, H. J. & Taylor, H. L. (1984). Measurement of physical activity in population studies: A review. *Human Biology, 56*, 195–216.

Myers, A. W. & Yeung, D. I. (1979). Obesity in infants: Significance, etiology, and prevention. *Canadian Journal of Public Health, 70*, 113–119.

O'Brien, T. P., Walley, P. B., Anderson-Smith, S., & Drabman, R. S. (1982). Naturalistic observation of the snack-selecting behavior of obese and non-obese children. *Addictive Behaviors, 7*, 75–77.

O'Neil, P. M., Currey, H. S., Malcolm, R., Francis, W.B., Riddle, F. E., & Sexaeur, J. D. (1982). Calorie counting by obese and non-obese subjects. *Obesity and Bariatric Medicine, 11*, 18–20.

Polivy, J. (1980). Restrained eating. In A. J. Stunkard (Ed.), *Obesity* (pp. 208–225). New York: Saunders.

Quay, H. & Werry, J. S. (1979). *Psychopathological Disorders of Childhood*(2nd ed.). New York: Wiley.

Sallade, J. A. (1973). Comparison of the psychological adjustment of obese vs. nonobese children. *Journal of Psychosomatic Research, 17*, 89–96.

Saltzstein, H. D. (1976). Social influence and moral development: A perspective on the role of parents and peers. In T. Lickona (Ed.), *Moral Development and Behavior*. NY: Holt, Rinehart, & Winston.

Schwartz, G. E. (1982). Testing the biopsychosocial model: The ultimate challenge facing behavioral medicine? *Journal of Consulting and Clinical Psychology, 50*, 1040–1053.

Shumaker, S. A. & Grunberg, N. (Eds.). (1986). Proceedings of the national working conference on smoking relapse. *Health Psychology, 5*(Suppl.), 1–99.

Staffieri, J.R. (1961). A study of social stereotypes of body image in children. *Journal of Personality and Social Psychology, 7*, 101–104.

Strauss, C.C., Smith K., Frame, C., & Forehand, R. (1985). Personal and interpersonal characteristics associated with childhood obesity. *Journal Pediatric Psychology, 10*, 337–343.

Streigel-Moore, R., & Rodin, J. (1986). The influence of psychological variables in obesity. In K. D. Brownell, & Foreyt, J. P. (Eds.), *Handbook of Eating Disorders: Physiology, Psychology, and Treatment of Obesity, Anorexia, and Bulimia*(pp. 99–121). NY: Basic Books.

Stunkard, A. J., & Mazer, A. (1978). Smorgasbord and obesity. *Psychosomatic Medicine, 40*, 173–175.

Stunkard, A. J. & Petska, J. (1962). The physical activity of obese girls. *American Journal of diseases in Children, 103*, 116–121.

Stunkard, A.J., Sorensen, T., Hanis, C., Teasdale, T.W., Chakraborty, R., Schull, W.J., & Schulsinger, F. (1986). An adoption study of human obesity. *New England Journal of Medicine, 314*, 193–198.

Stunkard, A. J. & Stellar, E. (Eds). (1984). *Eating and Its Disorders*. N.Y.: Raven.

Stunkard, A. J. & Waxman, M. (1981). Accuracy of self-reports of food intake. *Journal of the American Dietetic Association, 79*, 547-551.

Van Itallie, T. B. (1984). The enduring storage capacity for fat: Implications of obesity. In A. J. Stunkard & E. Stellar (Eds.), *Eating and Its Disorders*. New York: Raven.

Van Itallie, T.B. (1979). Obesity: Adverse effect on health and longevity. *American Journal of Clincial Nutrition, 32*, 2723–2733.

Volkmar, F. R., Stunkard, A. J., Woolston, J., & Bailey, R. J. (1981). High attrition rates in commercial weight reduction programs. *Archives of Internal Medicine, 141*, 426–428.

Waxman, M., & Stunkard, A. J. (1980). Caloric intake and expenditure of obese boys. *Journal of Pediatrics, 96, 187–193.*

Weber, J. M., Klesges, R. C., Suda, K., & Klesges, L. M. (in press) Chronic dieting and obesity: Their effects on dietary intake. *Journal of Behavioral Medicine.*

Weil, W. B. (1977). Current controversies in childhood obesity. *Journal of Pediatrics, 91,* 175–187.

Whitney, E. N. & Hamilton, E. M. N. (1984). *Understanding Nutrition* (3rd ed.). New York: West Publishing.

Wilkinson, P., Parklin, J., Pearloom, G., et al. (1977). Energy intake and physical activity in obese children. *British Medical Journal, 1,* 756.

Wooley, S. C., Wooley, O. W., & Dryenforth, S. R. (1979). Theoretical, practical, and social issues in behavioral treatment of obesity. *Journal of Applied Behavior Analysis, 12,* 3–25.

Zahn-Waxler, C., Radke-Yarrow, M., & King, R.A. (1979). Child-rearing and children's prosocial initiations toward victims of distress. *Child Development, 50,* 319–330.

Author Notes

This chapter was developed from a paper presented at the NICHD Workshop on Childhood Obesity, March 10–11, 1986, Bethesda, MD. This research was supported by grants from the National Heart, Lung, and Blood Institute (HL36553) and the National Institute of Child Health and Human Development (HD21330). Support was also received by a Centers of Excellence grant awarded to the Department of Psychology, Memphis State University, by the State of Tennessee.

III

PREVENTION

8

Physical Activity and Prevention of Obesity in Childhood

DEBRA G. CLARK AND STEVEN N. BLAIR
Division of Epidemiology
Institute For Aerobics Research
Dallas, Texas

The primary purpose of this chapter is to address the issue of whether sedentary living patterns cause or exacerbate obesity in childhood. The etiology of obesity is complex and can be related to genetic, hormonal and metabolic factors (Rabinowitz, 1970; Seltzer, 1969; Van Itallie, 1977). Yet, in a simplistic view, excessive food intake relative to caloric expenditure creates the energy imbalance that is responsible for excessive adiposity (Braunstein, 1971; Bray, 1983; Bullen et al., 1964; Chirico and Stunkard, 1960; Johnson et al., 1956; Mayer and Stare, 1953). It is generally accepted that exercise habits are somehow related to body composition, but the specific role of exercise is poorly documented. Participants in exercise training studies tend to lose body fat (Wilmore et al., 1970) and more physically active individuals in population studies are leaner (Buskirk and Taylor, 1957). What is not known is the specific mechanisms by which exercise may affect body composition. Is it simply a question of increased caloric expenditure via exercise, or are more complex factors involved? Does exercise help regulate appetite, and thus influence caloric intake as well as caloric expenditure? Is basal metabolic rate changed by exercise? The main question addressed in this chapter is whether the lack of exercise is a precursor to the development of obesity in children.

In addition to the main question stated above, we also address important ancillary issues that need resolution. For example, accurate and practical techniques should be developed for clinical assessment of body composition in children, and much work is needed on physical activity assessment methodology. In addition, the interactive role of exercise, diet, and other health habits needs to be elucidated. Finally, we will make recommendations for further study. For this paper, we reviewed published papers, examined some unpublished data from a national survey of health-related physical fitness in a representative sample of school children, and analyzed some of our existing data on physical fitness and adiposity.

I. Literature Review

A. Obesity as a Health Problem

1. *Adults.* Obesity is acknowledged as a health hazard due to its association with diabetes, hyperlipidemia, gallbladder disease, cardiovascular disease, and possible development of breast and endometrial carcinoma in women (Kannel and Gordon, 1974a; Kannel and Gordon, 1974b; Kannel et al., 1967; Keys, 1975; Keys et al., 1972; Mann, 1974; Rimm et al., 1972; Sims, 1979; USPHS, 1966; Van Itallie, 1979; Van Itallie, 1977). Reports from the Framingham Study indicate that being overweight is an independent coronary risk factor (Gordon and Kannel, 1973; Hubert et al., 1983).

2. *Children and adolescents.* Obesity is strongly associated with coronary risk factors in children and adolescents. It is clear that early attention to risk factors is important. Postmortem examinations were performed on young men (mean age 22 years) who were battle casualities during the Korean and Vietnam military conflicts. These examinations revealed a prevalence of atherosclerotic plaque on the aorta in 45% to 75% of the cases (Enos et al, 1953; McNamara et al., 1971). A prevalence rate this high in young men supports the hypothesis for early development of coronary heart disease in young people. Obesity in children and adolescents is associated with hyperinsulinemia, hypertension, decreased growth hormone secretion, and carbohydrate intolerance (Chiumello et al., 1969; Clarke et al., 1970; Court et al., 1974; Cronk et al., 1983; de Castro et al., 1976; Frerichs et al., 1978; Gilliam and Burke, 1978; Lauer et al., 1975, Londe et al., 1971, Martin and Martin, 1973; Stine et al., 1975). Recent cross-sectional studies indicate positive relationships between obesity and serum total cholesterol, serum triglycerides, and low-density lipoprotein-cholesterol (LDL-C) in children (Frerichs et al., 1978; Glueck et al., 1980, Laskarzewski et al., 1980; Orchard et al., 1981). In addition, an inverse relationship between high-density lipoprotein-cholesterol (HDL-C) and obesity has been reported (Frerichs et al., 1978; Glueck

et al., 1980; Laskarzewski et al., 1980, Newman et al., 1986, Orchard et al., 1981). A recent longitudinal study found positive associations between changes in triceps skinfold thickness and serum lipid levels (Freedman et al., 1985). Blood lipid levels are known to be associated with risk of coronary heart disease in adults; but until recently lipid levels in children were not shown to be associated with atherosclerosis. An autopsy study on teenagers and young adults in the Bogalusa Heart Study who died unexpectedly has now shown that blood lipids early in life are important (Newman et al., 1986). Total cholesterol and LDL-C levels obtained in infancy and childhood were positively associated with fatty streaks in the coronary arteries of teenagers and young adults up to ten years later.

Childhood obesity can have long-term detrimental effects on psychological development as well as on physiological factors. For example, obese individuals may be tagged with undesirable behavorial characteristics, such as social deviance and excessive self-gratification patterns. Due to the rapid growth and development occurring biologically and psychologically children are especially susceptible to adverse environmental effects (Johnston, 1985).

B. Tracking of Obesity into Adulthood

In childhood, the normal development of adipose tissue involves two stages. The first is marked by a rapid increase in adiposity during the first year of life due to the growth in adipose cell size (this growth rate diminishes in the next year or two and remains stable for the next two to three years). The second stage involves both an increase in the size and number of adipose cells and is termed the adiposity rebound (Hager et al., 1977; Knittle et al., 1979). The second stage of adiposity growth begins near the sixth year of life. Rolland-Cachera et al. (1984) suggest that excessive multiplication of adipocytes with an early adiposity rebound is more prevalent in obese children. Obese children demonstrate accelerated tissue development and growth (Bonnet and Lefebvre, 1977; Bonnet and Rocour-Brumioul, 1981; Forbes, 1977). Children that grow and develop at a faster rate than normal exhibit a significantly higher adiposity level (Rolland-Cachera et al., 1984). Bruch (1940), through observation of 140 case studies of children, noted that a rapidly growing child requires a greater amount of energy than a slowly growing child or an adult. Apparently obese children develop at a faster rate than nonobese children; therefore, the energy needs of obese children may exceed that of nonobese children.

There are risks associated with obesity in adults that should be recognized and addressed in childhood. Previously mentioned studies concerning postmortem examinations and other findings indicate that untreated risk factors in children will continue into adulthood (Clarke et al., 1978; Linder and Durant, 1982; Orchard et al., 1983). It is evident that coronary heart disease is both a pediatric (Blumenthal, 1973; Garn and La Velle, 1985; Kannel, 1976; Kannel and Dawber, 1972; Zack et al., 1979) and an adult problem.

The probability of an individual's becoming obese as an adult is greater if the individual was obese as a child. In addition, the probability of remaining obese as an adult becomes even greater as obese children become obese adolescents. However, not all obese children become obese adults nor are all obese adults a by-product of childhood obesity (Rolland-Cachera et al., 1984). In a study of two cycles of the U.S. Health Examination Survey, Zack et al. (1979) concluded that childhood fatness was highly predictive of adolescent fatness. In a longitudinal study of adolescents, Huenemann et al. (1974), found that individuals who were obese at age 14 tended to remain obese through ages 17 and 18. However, Braddon et al. (1986), in a 36-year birth cohort study, found the predictive value of childhood obesity to be minimal. Braddon found that 21.4% of this cohort who were obese at age 11 were also obese at age 36, whereas 78.6% first became obese in early adult life. Braddon states that there may be a post-war cohort effect on birthweight status due to food rationing. Since obesity can begin in childhood, it is important to recognize the associations between persistent obesity (specifically in children and adolescents), relative health risks, and the role of physical activity.

C.   Assessment of Physical Activity and Body Composition

Study of the role of physical activity as it relates to the development of obesity is hampered by a lack of valid and reliable assessment methods. Although most are imprecise, there are numerous techniques available for assessment of physical activity levels in children and adolescents. Self-administered questionnaires have been used to assess physical activity patterns (5- and 11-year follow-ups, work and/or leisure time activity questionnaires, activity self-rating questionnaires, 24-hour recall) (Baecke et al., 1982; Baranowski et al., 1984; Bouchard et al., 1983; Bradfield et al., 1971; Bullen et al., 1964; Durant et al., 1983; Engstrom, 1980; Kannel and Sorlie, 1979, O'Connell et al., 1985; Taylor et al., 1978; Wallace et al., 1985; Worsley et al., 1984). In addition, physical activity in children has been assessed through motion picture photography, pedometers, 24-hour recall, observation, interviews (parents and/or children), heart rate monitoring, oxygen consumption, and various methods of energy expenditure estimation (Bouchard et al., 1983, Bradfield et al., 1971, Bullen et al., 1964, Hovell et al., 1978, Johnson et al., 1956, LaPorte et al., 1982, Maxfield and Konishi, 1966; Stefanik et al., 1959; Stunkard and Pestka, 1962; Wallace et al., 1985, Waxman and Stunkard, 1980; Wilkinson et al., 1977). Self-administered questionnaires and other methods have been applied to summer camp settings, school-year-based settings, and/or both settings (Stefanik et al., 1959, Stunkard and Pestka, 1962). In addition, activities at leisure and school for obese and nonobese individuals have been investigated. Several studies on current physical activity participation in children are available, but the literature on long-term physical activity habit patterns is meager (Baecke et al., 1982; Bouchard et al., 1983; Bullen et al., 1964; Lauer et al., 1975). The various investigations differ in their conclusions concerning physical activity levels of obese children and adolescents versus nonobese children and adolescents. The methodology used in assessing regular physical activity in children and adolescents is still in the developmental stage and may lack the reliability and validity to ensure consistent and accurate data. This may be especially true when addressing obese children and adolescents or their parents/guardians. Obese children, adolescents, and/ or parents/guardians may judge physical activity differently from their nonobese counterparts. Still, the use of self-administered questionnaires or self-reported data is a practical approach for epidemiologic studies. Kohl et al. (1986) found a strong correlation (multiple $R=0.65$) between self-reported physical activity data and physical fitness level in a mail survey in an adult population. In addition, Ross and Gilbert (1985) found a significant association between mile run times and self-reported physical activity in an interview survey in children and adolescents. The use of an objective measure such as physical fitness as a surrogate (proxy) measure of physical activity offers an alternative to self-reported data with children and adolescents.

Lohman et al. recently reviewed body composition assessment methodology in children and adolescents (Lohman, 1981; Lohman, 1982; Lohman et al., 1984). Skinfold techniques have been widely used, and probably provide a useful index of body composition. However, technical issues such as chemical immaturity in prepubescent and adolescent children complicate estimation of body density and body composition. Further work is needed to provide better estimates of body composition and to define obesity in children.

D.   Role of Physical Activity in Obesity

1. *Adults.*   The role of physical activity in obesity is a complex issue that poses a challenging and important question. Does inactivity cause obesity, perpetuate obesity, result from obesity, or is it unrelated to obesity? As early as 1940, Rony observed a tendency for obese individuals to be less active than nonobese. In a study of adult workers, Mayer et al. (1956) classified the individuals according to the physical intensity of their jobs, into five groups, ranging from sedentary (low intensity) to very heavy (high intensity). The physical intensity of the job was inversely proportional to total body weight. Caloric intake had a J-shaped relationship to the job activity and was higher among the most active and most sedentary individuals (Mayer et al. 1956). The higher weights among the sedentary individuals may indicate that a moderate level of activity may be necessary in order to regulate caloric intake to match caloric expenditure. Bloom and Eidex (1976) found that obese adults spent significantly more time in bed or sitting than nonobese adults. As measured by self report (Mayer, et al., 1956; Rand and Stunkard, 1974), pedometers (Chirico and Stunkard, 1960), using stairs versus escalators (Brownell et al., 1980), and measuring standing versus sitting (Bloom and Eidex, 1967), obese adults are less active than nonobese adults. Apparently voluntary physical activity is low for obese individuals.

2. *Children and Adolescents.*   There are few studies of infant or early childhood activity levels; however, two studies report that heavier infants are less active than their lighter counterparts (Rose and Mayer, 1968; Mack and Kleinhenz, 1974). A longitudinal study from birth to early childhood indicated that there is no significant cross-sectional relationship between neonatal activity levels and neonatal adiposity levels; however, childhood activity levels during the daytime are significantly cross-sectionally associated with childhood adiposity levels (Berkowitz et al., 1985). Parizkova et al. (1986) examined a group of pre-school children and found that the highly active children (n=8) had lower body weight and fatness and better cardiorespiratory fitness than their inactive counterparts (n=9). The height of the children did not differ, but the body weight of the inactive children was 5% higher and the fatness 12% higher than the active children.

Numerous studies have shown that obese children and adolescents are less active than their nonobese counterparts (Bullen et al., 1964; Johnson et al., 1956; Stefanik et al., 1959; Waxman and Stunkard, 1980). Using questionnaires, interviews, and personal visits, Bruch (1940) collected relevant information on 140 obese children. Of those 140 case studies, Bruch found 66% of the boys and 68% of the girls to be physically inactive. Eighteen percent of the boys and 22.5% of the girls demonstrated normal activity patterns. The remaining children reported inconsistent behavior patterns that were regarded as both inactive and normal from a day-to-day basis. Though most of the obese children were inactive, Bruch found no apparent association between activity levels and degree of obesity. Johnson et al. (1956) found that obese high school girls were less active than nonobese girls. Other studies suggest that the activity level of obese children and adolescents is similar to that of the nonobese, yet the obese expend the same or a greater amount of energy during a 24-hour period due to greater total body mass (Bradfield et al., 1971; Maxfield and Konishi, 1966; Stunkard and Pestka, 1962; Wilkinson et al., 1977).

There are a few exercise training experiments involving children and adolescents, and the results are generally the same as similar studies involving adults (Malina, 1984; Parizkova, 1977). The training groups tend to increase in lean body mass and decrease in body fat. Malina (1984) indicated that regular exercise plays an important role in the maintenance of body weight, but that results are inconsistent across studies. Malina also reviewed the impact of exercise directly upon adipose tissue. He concluded that the impact of exercise, sex differences, and developmental trends on regional variability in adipose cell number and size is not consistent across the published studies.

Rolland-Cachera et al. (1984) noted that an early adiposity rebound may identify children at a greater risk of becoming obese. Identification of children who may become obese adults is important, yet we must still address the issues related to the mechanisms that affect body composition. In essence, without addressing the complexities involved, obesity results from energy intake in excess of energy expenditure. Rolland-Cachera et al. (1984) suggest that the development of excess adipose tissue might be due to genetic factors, hormonal factors, or energy imbalance. The actual causes of obesity are those factors that foster excessive energy intake, reduce energy expenditure, or impair the regulation of energy balance (Dietz, 1983). The measurement of daily energy expenditure and energy cost during specific activities can provide insight into the complex relationship between physical activity and childhood obesity. Total daily energy expenditure is determined by basal energy expenditure and muscular activity. A major determinant of basal metabolic rate is the amount of lean body mass, and it is generally accepted that higher levels of obesity are associated with increased levels of lean body mass (Dietz, 1983; Miller and Blyth, 1953). Therefore, obese children and adolescents have basal metabolic rates that are equivalent to or higher than nonobese children and adolescents. (Dietz, 1983; James et al., 1978). Total daily energy expenditure is also determined by the total amount of muscular activity performed, and, as shown above, the obese are generally more inactive. Therefore, the obese may expend more energy via basal processes, but less via voluntary muscular activity. The net effect may be that the total energy expenditure may be the same in obese and nonobese.

The issue of energy balance is further complicated by addressing dietary habits. Dietary studies comparing obese children and adolescents with nonobese children and adolescents yield differing results, with some researchers finding lower caloric intake among the obese (Johnson et al., 1956; Stefanik et al., 1959). Other studies have found the same or a higher caloric intake among the obese (Maxfield and Konishi, 1966; Perusse et al., 1984; Wilkinson et al., 1977). One must also consider the seasonal variation associated with both physical activity and diet, and not all studies have accounted for this effect (Dotson and Ross, 1985; Stefanik et al., 1959).

II. Current Studies

A. National Children and Youth Fitness Study (NCYFS)

The Office of Disease Prevention and Health Promotion, an agency of the U.S. Public Health Service, commissioned a nationwide study on health related physical fitness in 5th through 12th grade students (NCYFS) in 1984. A national probability sample of more than 10,000 children was drawn with approximately 85% (8,800 students) of the sample participating in the survey. Data collected included demographic information, a physical activity survey, and physical fitness items. The physical fitness items were primarily taken from the American Alliance for Health, Physical Education, Recreation, and Dance (AAHPERD) Health Related Physical Fitness Test (HRPFT) (AAHPERD 1980). Physical fitness test items discussed in this paper are cardiorespiratory endurance (assessed by the one mile run/walk) and body composition (assessed by triceps and subscapular skinfolds). Summary results from the survey have been published (Ross and Gilbert, 1985), but additional unpublished data were used for this report (courtesy of James Ross, Macro Systems).

These analyses examined the relationship between physical activity habits, body composition, and cardiorespiratory endurance. The physical activity survey data were used to identify students who engaged in appropriate levels of physical activity (defined as exercise involving large muscle groups, for 20 minutes or more, three or more times weekly, at an intensity of at least 60% of maximal cardiorespiratory capacity). An index of physical activity was constructed by indicating the number of seasons in which a student participated in appropriate physical activity (0-4 seasons). Multiple linear regression analyses (SAS, 1985) were done with skinfolds as the dependent variables and physical activity index, age, and sex (and their interaction terms) as independent variables. Least squares means for skinfolds by physical activity categories were also calculated.

The data from NCYFS analyses are presented in Table 1. Although these preliminary analyses should be interpreted cautiously, there is a trend for lower skinfold values in the more active children. The apparent impact of activity is more pronounced in the most inactive children. This may indicate a threshold of physical activity necessary to maintain appropriate body composition.

A second analysis from the NCYFS showed a highly significant trend for mile run/walk time across the physical activity strata. Mean mile run times (minutes) were 10.6, 10.5, 10.1, 9.9, and 9.5 across the activity strata (0-4 respectively). This highly significant trend ($p < 0.0001$) supports the use of cardiorespiratory fitness measures as a marker for appropriate physical activity.

B.   FITNESSGRAM

The Institute for Aerobics Research (IAR) has established a large database of student physical fitness scores through the development and delivery of FITNESSGRAM. FITNESSGRAM is a nationwide computerized system for assessing and reporting physical fitness levels of school children (grades K-12) (Weber et al., 1986). The FITNESSGRAM

Table I

Least squares means* for skinfold measures by physical activity status in the NCYFS.

	Skinfolds (mm)	
Physical Activity Index +	Triceps	Subscapular
0	14.0[‡]	11.5[‡]
1	13.4	10.8
2	13.2	10.5
3	13.6	10.3
4	13.1	10.4

* Adjusted for sex, age, and interactions
+ Index is number of seasons engaging in appropriate physical activity
‡ Significant difference across activity groups $p < 0.0001$

data reported here are from the AAHPERD HRPFT (AAHPERD, 1980). The test battery was administered to school children by physical education instructors. The results of individual student performance are documented on a report card (FITNESSGRAM) which is sent to each student's parents/guardians. The FITNESSGRAM evaluation provides direct feedback to the students, parents, teachers, and school administrators regarding individual and group/class physical fitness status. FITNESSGRAM was initiated in the fall of 1982 in a single city, expanded to statewide delivery the following year, and nationwide delivery in 1984.

In this paper we examined 1985−86 FITNESSGRAM data from the HRPFT test battery (ages 5−17 years), which was administered to 18,141 students (9,050 males and 9,091 females) in 18 school districts in 13 states. The HRPFT provides options for the individual teacher for test administration of the adiposity measure and cardiorespiratory measure. The variables examined included three indices of adiposity and four measures of cardiorespiratory fitness. In our analyses we used cardiorespiratory fitness as a marker for physical activity. The measurement of physical fitness (cardiorespiratory fitness) is an objective, reliable, valid, and practical assessment method. Accurate self-reported physical activity data are difficult to obtain in children and youth. They have problems remembering the specific activities in which they participated during the past week. Furthermore, they have even more difficulty in estimating the time spent in specific activities. Therefore, using cardiorespiratory fitness as a marker for physical activity habits is a reasonable alternative.

Some have argued that the correlation between physical activity and physical fitness is low, and in most reports the correlation coefficients are about 0.3-0.5. However, more recent studies in adults show higher correlations (multiple R = 0.65) (Kohl et al., 1986). In unpublished analyses, we find correlations between fitness and activity in adults to range from 0.66 to 0.83 in various age and sex groups. In these latter studies, the physical activity was determined from a historical record. These data were from individuals who self-reported their physical activity after each exercise bout. Data analysis was performed on individuals who had recorded their exercise activities for six months prior to a maximal treadmill test. Thus, when a more complete record of physical activity is used, relatively high correlations are seen with objectively determined physical fitness. In the NCYFS, data on habitual physical activity and physical fitness were collected. Physical fitness as measured by time for the one mile walk/run and habitual physical activity as measured by self-report were positively associated in children and adolescents (Ross and Gilbert, 1985). Physical fitness not only serves as a marker for physical activity, but there is a dose response relationship between physical activity and physical fitness (Fox et al., 1975; Gettman et al., 1976).

In our analysis of the FITNESSGRAM data we examined three measures of adiposity which included body mass index ((BMI), BMI=Weight (Kg)/ Height $(M)^2$), triceps skinfold measurement, and triceps plus subscapular skinfold measurement. All students have a BMI measurement, some of these students have a triceps skinfold measurement (3,320 males and 3,817 females), and a subset of this latter group also have subscapular skinfold measurements. The triceps plus subscapular skinfold group has 1,730 males and 2,327 females. Individual students may have more than one measure of adiposity, but each student will have only one measure of cardiorespiratory fitness. Cardiorespiratory fitness was assessed through one of four running tests (1 mile, 1.5 mile, 9 minute or 12 minute). To simplify analyses and permit pooling of data from the various cardiorespiratory fitness tests, all four running test scores were algebraically transformed into a velocity variable (feet/second). A preliminary analysis of a sample of FITNESSGRAM participants found essentially identical mean velocity scores for the four running tests within each age and sex group.

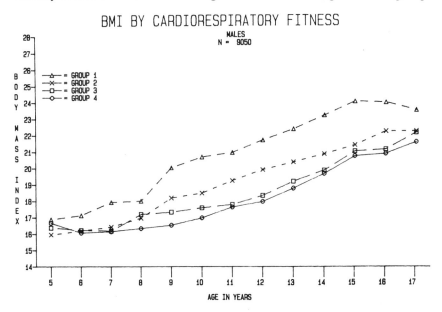

Figure 1. Mean scores for body mass index by cardiorespiratory fitness group by age for males in FITNESSGRAM. Groups represent cardiorespiratory fitness quartiles. GROUP 1 = 0–25% tile (least fit); GROUP 2 = 26–50% tile; GROUP 3 = 51–75% tile; GROUP 4 = 76+% tile.

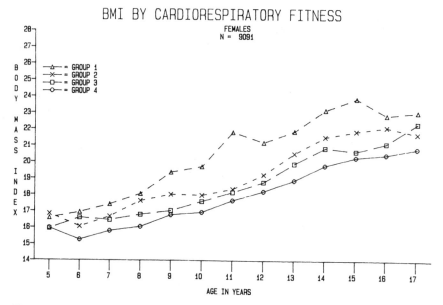

Figure 2. Mean scores for body mass index by cardiorespiratory fitness group by age for females in FITNESSGRAM. Groups represent cardiorespiratory fitness quartiles. GROUP 1 = 0–25% tile (least fit); GROUP 2 = 26–50% tile; GROUP 3 = 51–75% tile; GROUP 4 = 76+% tile.

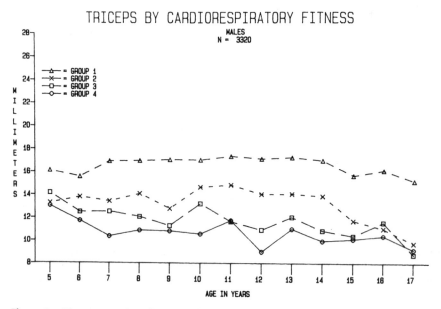

Figure 3. Mean scores for triceps skinfold by cardiorespiratory fitness group by age for males in FITNESSGRAM. Groups represent cardiorespiratory fitness quartiles. GROUP 1 = 0–25% tile (least fit); GROUP 2 = 26–50% tile; GROUP 3 = 51–75% tile; GROUP 4 = 76+% tile.

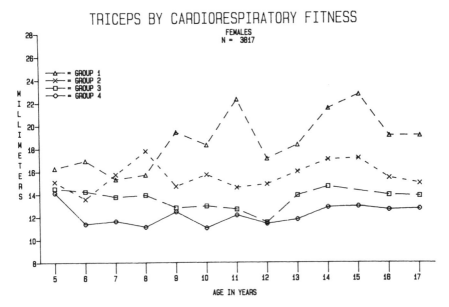

Figure 4. Mean scores for triceps skinfold by cardiorespiratory fitness group by age for females in FITNESSGRAM. Groups represent cardiorespiratory fitness quartiles. GROUP 1 = 0–25% tile (least fit); GROUP 2 = 26–50% tile; GROUP 3 = 51–75% tile; GROUP 4 = 76+% tile.

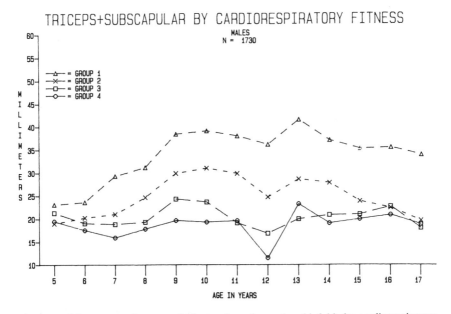

Figure 5. Mean scores for sum of triceps plus subscapular skinfolds by cardiorespiratory fitness group by age for males. Groups represent cardiorespiratory fitness quartiles. GROUP 1 = 0–25% tile (least fit); GROUP 2 = 26–50% tile; GROUP 3 = 51–75% tile; GROUP 4 = 76+% tile.

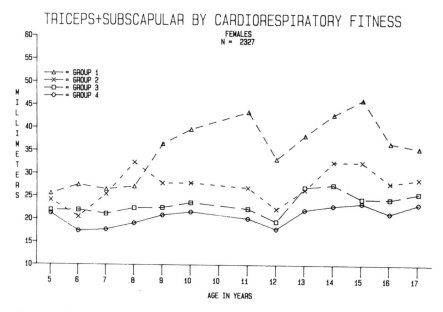

Figure 6. Mean scores for sum of triceps plus subscapular skinfolds by cardiorespiratory fitness group by age for females. Groups represent cardiorespiratory fitness quartiles. GROUP 1 = 0–25% tile (least fit); GROUP 2 = 26–50% tile; GROUP 3 = 51–75% tile; GROUP 4 = 76+% tile.

The similar distributions for the four running tests gave us confidence that the velocity scores could be pooled in further analyses. Based on velocity scores the students were classified into fitness quartiles (Group 1 = 0–25% tile; Group 2 = 26–50% tile; Group 3 = 51–75% tile; Group 4 = 76+% tile). In order to examine the relationship between cardiorespiratory fitness and adiposity, the mean adiposity values were computed by fitness group, by age and by sex.

The mean adiposity values by age for each fitness group were plotted for males and females for each of the adiposity measures (Figures 1-6). Each of the graphs shows an inverse relationship between adiposity level and cardiorespiratory fitness. An analysis of variance was performed using adiposity level as the dependent variable, fitness group as the factor, and covarying for age and sex. The main effect of fitness group was significant (p < 0.0001) for all three adiposity measures indicating that the inverse relationships between cardiorespiratory fitness and adiposity apparent on the graphs are statistically significant.

The relationships between the three adiposity measures and cardiorespiratory fitness groups across the age range are consistent in both males and females. There is an ordered association with the least fit being the fattest and the most fit the leanest. The effect is most noticable for the lowest quartile fitness group for both sexes and for all adiposity measures. Further, analyses of variance showed that the least fit group was significantly ($p < 0.0001$) fatter than the other three fitness groups combined. The adiposity-fitness group relationship is less pronounced at the youngest and the oldest age groups in some of the analyses. This is probably due to instability caused by small sample sizes in the most extreme age groups.

III. Conclusions

Our primary purpose was to address the issue of whether or not sedentary living patterns cause or exacerbate obesity in childhood. We gave particular attention to the question of whether the lack of exercise precedes the development of obesity in children. The literature review provides the following summary points:

Obesity is a health hazard for children, adolescents, and adults.
Obesity tracks into adulthood.
Coronary risk factors associated with obesity track into adulthood.
Obese children are less active than nonobese children
Adiposity measurement is somewhat imprecise, but nonetheless useful.
Physical fitness is inversely related to adiposity.
Regular activity can contribute to decreased adiposity levels, disease prevention, and improved health status.

Analyses of two large national databases on physical fitness in children and adolescents confirms and extends findings from previous studies. The strength of these analyses is that large representative samples of students were available for study. Most of the published reports are on relatively small and select samples. The NCYFS provides for the first time data on habitual activity patterns and body composition in males and females across a broad age range in a large and representative sample. These data suggest a strong relationship between physical activity and obesity. The NCYFS also provides evidence on the validity of using cardiorespiratory fitness data as a marker for habitual physical activity patterns. Since objective measures of cardiorespiratory fitness are much easier to obtain than estimates of physical activity level, large scale studies can be more efficiently conducted using cardiorespiratory fitness tests as surrogate measures of exercise patterns.

The FITNESSGRAM analyses further support a strong link between physical activity, physical fitness, and adiposity. The associations were strong, graded, and consistent across age and sex groups and for the different measures of adiposity. The association between fitness groups and adiposity was most notable in the lowest fitness quartile of students. This may suggest a threshold level of physical activity for normal body composition in children and adolescents. That is, only the most inactive have a greater prevalence of obesity. The graded association of adiposity across the top three quartiles of fitness is less striking and may well be confounded by genetic factors and complex physiological and biomechanical factors related to running. A graded effect of habitual physical activity and adiposity was demonstrated in the NCYFS data. In addition, the least active group had proportionally greater skinfold measurements when adjacent physical activity groups were compared (J.G. Ross, Macro Systems, unpublished data). These NCYFS data provide further support for our speculation that there may be a threshold of physical activity (physical fitness) appropriate for the maintenance of normal body composition.

Our review strongly suggests an association between physical activity and adiposity in children and adolescents. All studies reviewed have serious limitations such as small sample size, cross-sectional design, short-term follow-up, or inadequate assessment of key variables. Our own analyses are cross-sectional and therefore limited. It is premature to conclude that there is a cause and effect relationship between sedentary habits and the development of obesity in children and youth. The complex cause and effect relationship associated with the development of childhood obesity involves the consideration of many factors including nutritional factors, genetic predisposition, physical activity, and/or a combination of many factors.

IV. Recommendations

Additional studies are needed, and can be enhanced by more methodological work on assessment of physical activity patterns and body composition. The continued development of questionnaires for assessing physical activity in children and adolescents and further work with physical fitness assessment as a surrogate measure of physical activity require additional research. The use of physical fitness offers an objective and reliable method, but still requires further consideration. The interaction of diet and physical activity also needs more research.

In order to provide data on the primary question on the causal relationship between sedentary living patterns and the development of obesity, prospective studies must be undertaken. Careful assessments of physical fitness, physical activity, and body composition must be obtained on a large representative sample of children; and these children must be followed for several years. Careful and complete monitoring of the development of obesity in this cohort must be done. These studies should include children of various ages, but must include some young children of nursery school age at baseline.

Acknowledgments

We thank Harold W. Kohl, M.S.P.H. for his assistance in data analysis, the Division of Computer Services for program development and continued support, Marilu D. Meredith Ed.D. for technical assistance, and David Moorefield for research assistance.

This research is supported by a grant from the Campbell Soup Company.

References

American Alliance for Health, Physical Education, Recreation, and Dance. (1980) *AAHPERD* Health Related Physical Fitness Test Manual. Reston, Virginia: AAHPERD.

Baecke, J. A. H., Burema, J., & Frijters, J. E. R. (1982). A short questionnaire for the measurement of habitual physical activity in epidemiological studies. *Am. J. Clin. Nutr.,* *36*, 936–941.

Baranowski, T., Dworkin, R. J., Cieslik, C. J., Hooks, P., Clearman, D. R., Ray, L., Dunn, J. K., & Nader, P. R. (1984). Reliability and validity of self report of aerobic activity: Family health project. *Res. Quart. Ex. Sport.,* *55(4)*, 309–317.

Berkowitz, R. I., Agras, W. S., Korner, A. F., Kraemer, H. C., & Zeanah, C. H. (1985). Physical activity and adiposity: A longitudinal study from birth to childhood. *J. Pediatrics,* *106(5)*, 734–738.

Bloom, W. L., & Eidex, M. F. (1967). Inactivity as a major factor in adult obesity. *Metabolism,* *16*, 679–684.

Blumenthal, S. (1973). Prevention of atherosclerosis. *Am. J. Cardiol.,* *31*, 591–594.

Bonnet, F., & Lefebvre, P. (1977). Prevention chez l'enfant de l'obesite de l'adulte. *Med. Nutr.,* *13*, 15–21.

Bonnet, F. P., & Rocour-Brumioul, D. (1981). Normal growth of human adipose tissue. In: *Adipose tissue in childhood (Eds: Fernand and Bonnet) Boca Raton*, Florida: CRC Press Inc, pp. 81–107.

Bouchard, C., Tremblay, A., Leblanc, C., Lortie, G., Savard, R., & Theriault, G. (1983). A method to assess energy expenditure in children and adults. *Am. J. Clin. Nutr.,* *37*, 461–467.

Braddon, F. E. M., Rodgers, B., Wadsworth, M. E. J., & Davies, J. M. C. (1986). Onset of obesity in a 36 year birth cohort study. *Brit. Med. J.,* *293*, 299–303.

Bradfield, R. B., Paulos, J., & Grossman, L. (1971). Energy expenditure and heart rate of obese high school girls. *Am. J. Clin. Nutr.,* *24*, 1482–1488.

Braunstein, J. J. (1971). Management of the obese patient. *Med. Clin. North. Am.*, *55(2)*, 391–401.

Bray, G. A. (1983) The energetics of obesity. *Med. Sci. Sports.*, *15(1)*, 32–40.

Brownell, K. D., Stunkard, A. J., & Albaum, J. M. (1980). Evaluation and modification of activity patterns in the natural environment. *Amer. J. Psychiat.*, *137(12)*, 1540–1545.

Bruch, H. (1940). Obesity in childhood. IV. Energy expenditure of obese children. *Am. J. Dis. Child.*, *59*, 1082–1109.

Bullen, B. A., Reed, R. B., & Mayer, J. (1964). Physical activity of obese and non obese adolescent girls appraised by motion picture sampling. *Am. J. Clin. Nutr.*, *14*, 211–223.

Buskirk, E. R., & Taylor, H. L. (1957). Maximal oxygen uptake and it relation to body composition, with special reference to chronic physical activity and obesity. *J. Appl. Physiol.*, *11*, 72–78.

Chirico, A., & Stunkard, A. J. (1960). Physical activity and human obesity. *New Engl. J. Med.*, *263*, 935–940.

Chiumello, G., Del Guercio, M. J., Cornelutti, M., & Bidme, G. (1969). Relationship between obesity, chemical diabetes, and beta-pancreatic function in children. *Diabetes*, *18*, 238.

Clarke, R. P., Morrow, S. B., & Morse, E. H. (1970). Interrelationships between plasma lipids, physical measurements, and body fatness of adolescents in Burlington, Vermont. *Am. J. Clin. Nutr.*, *23*, 754–763.

Clarke, W. R., Schrott, H. E., Leaverton, P. E., Connor, W. E., & Lauer, R. M. (1978). Tracking of blood lipids and blood pressure in school aged children: The Muscatine study. *Circulation*, *58(4)*, 624–633.

Court, J. M., Hill, G. J., Dunlop, M., & Boulton, T. J. C. (1974). Hypertension in childhood obesity. *Aust. Paediatr. J.*, *10*, 296–300.

Cronk, C. E., Roche, A. F., Kent, R., Eichorn, D., & McCammon, R. W. (1983). Longitudinal trends in subcutaneous fat thickness during adolescence. *Am. J. Phys. Anthrop.*, *61*, 197–204.

de Castro, F. J., Biesbroeck, R., Erikson, C., Farrell, P., Leong, W., Murphy, D., & Green, R. (1976). Hypertension in adolescents. *Clin. Pediatr.*, *15*, 24–26.

Dietz, W. H. (1983). Childhood obesity: Susceptibility, cause, and management. *J. Pediatrics*, *103(5)*, 676–685.

Dotson, C. O., & Ross, J. G. (1985). Relationships between activity patterns and fitness. *JOPHERD* (January), 86–90.

Durant, R. H., Linder, C. W., Harkess, J. W., & Gray, R. G. (1983). The relationship between physical activity and serum lipids and lipoproteins in black children and adolescents. *J. Adol. Hlth. Care.*, *4(1)*, 55–60.

Engstrom, L. M. (1980). Physical activity of children and youth. *Acta. Paediatr. Scand.*, *283*(suppl), 101–105.

Enos, W. F., Holmes, R. H., & Beyer, C. (1953). Coronary disease among United States soldiers killed in action in Korea: Preliminary report. *JAMA*, *152*, 1090–1093.

Forbes, G. B. (1977). Nutrition and growth. *J. Pediatrics*, *91(1)*, 40–42.

Fox, E. L., Bartels, R. L., Billings, C. E., O'Brien, R., Bason, R., & Mathews, D. K. (1975). Frequency and duration of interval training programs and changes in aerobic power. *J. Appl. Physiol.*, *38(3)*, 481–484.

Freedman, D. S., Burke, G. L., Harsha, D. W., Srinivasan, S. R., Cresanta, J. L., Webber, L. S., & Berenson, G. S. (1985). Relationship of changes in obesity to serum lipid and lipoprotein changes in childhood and adolescence. *JAMA*, *254(4)*, 515–520.

Frerichs, R. R., Webber, L. S., Srinivasan S. R., & Berenson G. S, (1978). Relation of serum lipids and lipoproteins to obesity and sexual maturation in white and black children. *Am. J. Epidemiol*, *108*, 486–496.

Garn, S. M., & La Velle, M., (1985). Two-decade follow-up of fatness in early childhood. *Am. J. Dis. Child.*, *139*, 181−185.

Gettman L. R., Pollock, M. L., Durstine, J. L., Ward, A., Ayres J., & Linnerud A. C. (1976). Physiological responses of men to 1, 3, and 5 day per week training programs. *Res. Quart.*, *47(4)*, 638−646.

Gilliam, T. B. & Burke, M. B. (1978). Effects of exercise on serum lipids and lipoproteins in girls, ages 8−10 years. *Artery*, *4*, 203−213.

Glueck, C. J., Taylor, H. L., Jacobs, D., Morrison, J. A., Beaglehole, R. & Williams, O. D. (1980). Plasma high-density lipoprotein cholesterol: Association with measurements of body mass: Lipid Research Clinics Program Prevalence Study. *Circulation*, *62*(suppl 4), 62−69.

Gordon, T., & Kannel, W. B. (1973). The effects of overweight on cardiovascular disease. *Geriatrics*, *28*, 80−88.

Hager, A., Sjostrom, L., Arvidsson, B., Bjorntorp, P., & Smith U. (1977). Body fat and adipose tissue cellularity in infants: A longitudinal study. *Metabolism*, *26(6)*, 607−614.

Hovell, M. F., Bursick, J. H., Sharkey, R., & McClure, J. (1978). An evaluation of elementary students' voluntary physical activity during recess. *Res. Quart*, *49*, 460−474.

Hubert, H. B., Feinleib, M., McNamara, P. M., & Castelli, W. P. (1983). Obesity as an independent risk factor for cardiovascular disease: A 26-year follow-up of participants in the Framingham Study. *Circulation*, *67(5)*, 968−977.

Huenemann, R. L., Hampton, M. C., Behnke, A. R., Shapiro, L. R., & Mitchell, B. W. (1974). *Teenage Nutrition and Physique*. Springfield, Illinois: Charles C. Thomas.

James, W. P. T., Davies, H. L., Bailes, J., & Dauncey, M. J. (1978). Elevated metabolic rates in obesity. *Lancet 1 (8074)*, 1122−1125.

Johnson, M. L., Burke, B. S., & Mayer, J. (1956). Relative importance of inactivity and overeating in the energy balance of obese high school girls. *Am. J. Clin. Nutr.*, *4(1)*, 37−43.

Johnston, F. E. (1985). Health implications of childhood obesity. *Annals of Int. Medicine*, *103(6:2)*, 1068−1072.

Kannel, W. B. (1976). Prospects for prevention of atherosclerosis in the young. *Aust. N. Z. J. Med.*, *6*, 410−419.

Kannel, W. B., & Dawber, T. R. (1972). Atherosclerosis as a pediatric problem. *J. Pediatr.*, *80*, 544−559.

Kannel, W. B., & Gordon T. (1974a). Obesity and cardiovascular disease: The Framingham Study. In: *Obesity* Burland, W., Samuel, P. D., Yudkin, J. (Eds.), London: Churchill Livingston.

Kannel, W. B., & Gordon, T. (1974b). The Framingham Study: An epidemiological investigation of cardiovascular disease, section 30. Some characteristics related to the incidence of cardiovascular disease and death: Framingham Study, 18-year follow-up. Washington, DC: U.S. Department of Health, Education and Welfare, Public Health Service, National Institutes of Health, DHEW Publication No. (NIH) 74−599.

Kannel, W. B., LeBauer, E. J., Dawber, T. R., & McNamara P. M. (1967). Relation of body weight to development of coronary heart disease: The Framingham Study. *Circulation*, *35*, 734−744.

Kannel, W. B., & Sorlie, P. (1979). Some health benefits of physical activity. *Arch. Intern. Med.*, *139(8)*, 857−861.

Keys, A. (1975). Coronary heart disease—the global picture. *Atherosclerosis*, *22*, 149.

Keys, A., Aravanis, C., Blackburn, H., Van Buchein F. S. P., Buzina, R., Djordjevic, B. S., Fdanza, F., Karvonen, M. J., Minottia, A., Puddu, V., & Taylor, H. L. (1972). Coronary heart disease: Overweight and obesity as risk factors. *Ann Intern Med.*, *77(1)*, 15−27.

Knittle, J. L., Timmers, K., Ginsberg-Fellner F. F., Brown R. E., & Katz, D. P. (1979). The growth of adipose tissue in children and adolescents. Cross-sectional and longitudinal studies of adipose cell number and size. *J. Clin. Invest.*, *63*, 239–246.

Kohl, H, W., Blair, S. N., & Paffenbarger, R. S., Jr. (1986). Validity of self report exercise habit responses in a mail survey. *Med. Sci. Sports Exercise*, *18(2)*, *Suppl: (abstract)*.

LaPorte, R. E., Cauley, J. A., Kinsey, C. M., Corbett, W., Robertson, R. Black-Sandler R., Kuller, L. H., & Falkel, J. (1982). The epidemiology of physical activity in children, college students, middle-aged men, menopausal females and monkeys. *J. Chron. Dis.*, *35*, 787–795.

Lauer, R. M., Conner, W. E., Leaverton, P. E., Reiter, M. A., & Clarke, W. R. (1975). Coronary heart disease risk factors in school children: The Muscatine Study. *J. Pediatr.*, *86*, 697–706.

Laskarzewski, P. M., Morrison, J. A., Mellies, M. J., Kelly, K., Gartside P. S., Khoury, P., & Glueck, C. J. (1980). Relationships of measurments of body mass to plasma lipoproteins in school children and adults. *Am. J. Epidemiol.*, *III(4)*, 395–406.

Linder, C. W., & Durant, R. H., (1982). Exercise, serum lipids, and cardiovascular disease-risk factors in children. *Pediatr. Clin. North Am.*, *29(6)*, 1341–1354.

Lohman, T. G. (1981). Skinfolds and body density and their relation to body fatness: A review. *Human Biology*, *53(2)*, 181–225.

Lohman, T. G. (1982). Measurements of body composition in children. *J. Phys. Ed. Rec.*, *53*, 67–70.

Lohman, T. G., Boileau, R. A., & Slaughter, M. H. (1984). Body composition in children and youth. In: *Advances in Pediatric Sports Sciences*. Boileau, R. A. (Ed.). *Human Kinetics*, 29–57.

Londe, S., Bourgoyne, J. J., Robson, A. M., & Goldring, D. (1971). Hypertension in apparently normal children. *J. Pediatr.*, *78*, 569–575.

Mack, R. W, & Kleinhenz, M. E. (1974). Growth, caloric intake, and activity levels of early infancy: A preliminary report. *Hum. Biol.*, *46*, 345.

Malina, R. M. (1984). Human growth, maturation, and regular physical activity. In: *Advances in Pediatric Sports Sciences*. Boileau, R. H. (Ed.). *Human Kinetics*, pp. 59–83.

Mann, G. V. (1974). The influence of obesity on health. *New England J. Med.*, *291*, 177–185.

Martin, M. M., & Martin A. L. A. (1973). Obesity, hyperinsulinism, and diabetes mellitus in childhood. *J. Pediatr.*, *82*, 192–201.

Maxfield, E., & Konishi, F. (1966). Patterns of food intake and physical activity in obesity. *J. Am. Diet. Assoc.*, *49*, 406–408.

Mayer, J., & Stare, F. (1953). Exercise and weight control. *J. Am. Diet. Accoc.*, *29*, 340–343.

Mayer, J. P., Roy, R., & Mitra, K. P. (1956). Relation between caloric intake, body weight, and physical work: Studies of an industrial male population in West Bengal. *Am. J. Clin. Nutrition*, *4*, 169–175.

McNamara, J. J., Molot, M. A., Stremple, J. F., & Cutting, R. T. (1971). Coronary artery disease in combat casualities in Vietnam. *JAMA*, *216*, 1185–1187.

Miller, A. T., & Blyth, C. S. (1953). Lean body mass as a metabolic reference standard. *J. Appl. Physiol.*, *5*, 311.

Newman, W. P., Freedman, D. S., Voors, A. W., Gard, P. D., Srinivasan, S. R., Cresanta, J. L., Williamson G. D., Webber L. S., & Berenson, G. S. (1986). Relation of serum lipoprotein levels and systolic blood pressure to early atherosclerosis. *New Engl. J. Med.*, *314(3)*, 138–144.

O'Connell J. K., Price, J. H., Roberts, S. M., Jurs, S. G., & McKinley, R. (1985). Utilizing the health belief model to predict dieting and exercising behavior of obese and nonobese adolescents. *Hlth. Ed. Quart.*, *12(4)*, 343–351.

Orchard, T. J., Rodgers M., Hedley, A. J., & Mitchell, J. R. (1981). Serum lipids in a teenage population: Geographic, seasonal, and familial factors. *Int. J. Epidemiol.*, *10(2)*, 161–170.

Orchard, T. J., Donahue, R. P., Kuller, L. H., Hodge P. N., & Drash, A. L. (1983). Cholesterol screening in childhood: Does it predict adult hypercholesterolemia? The Beaver County experience. *J. Pediatr.*, *103(5)*, 687–691.

Parizkova, J. (1977). *Body Fat and Physical Fitness*. The Hague: Martins, Nijhoff.

Parizkova, J., Mackova E., Kabele, J.. Mackova, J., & Skopkova, M. (1986). Body composition, food intake, cardiorespiratory fitness, blood lipids and psychological development in highly active and inactive preschool children. *Hum. Biol.*, *58(2)*, 261–273.

Perusse, L., Bouchard C., Leblanc, C. & Tremblay, A. (1984). Energy intake and physical fitness in children and adults of both sexes. *Nutr. Res.*, *4*, 363–370.

Rabinowitz, D. (1970). Some endocrine and metabolic aspects of obeisty. *Annu. Rev. Med.*, *21*, 241–258.

Rand, C., & Stunkard, A. J. (1974). Obesity and psychoanalysis. *Amer. J. Psychiat.*, *135*, 547–551.

Rimm, A. A., Werner, L. H., Bernstein, R., & VanYserloo, B. (1972). Disease and obesity in 73,532 women. *Obesity/Bariatric Med.*, *1*, 77–82.

Rolland-Cachera, M., Deheeger, M., Bellisle, F., Sempe', M., Guilloud-Bataille, & Patois, E. (1984). Adiposity rebound in children: A simple indicator for predicting obesity. *Am. J. Clin. Nutr.*, *39*, 129–135.

Rony, H. R. (1940). *Obesity and Leanness*. Philadelphia, PA: Lea & Febiger.

Rose, H. E, & Mayer, J. (1968). Activity, caloric intake, fat storage, and the energy balance of infants. *Pediatrics*, *41*, 18.

Ross, J. G, & Gilbert, G. G. (1985). A summary of findings. *JOPHERD (January)*, 45–50.

SAS Institute. (1985). *SAS user's guide: statistics. Version 5 edition*. Cary, NC: SAS.

Stefanik, P. A., Heald, F. P., & Mayer, J. (1959). Caloric intake in relation to energy output of obese and non-obese adolescent boys. *Am. J. Clin. Nutr.*, *7*, 55–61.

Seltzer, C. (1969). Genetics and obesity in physiopathology of adipose tissue. *Exerpta Med. Intl.*, J. Vague (Ed.) (p. 325).

Sims, E. A. H. (1979). Syndromes of obesity. In: *Endocrinology*, DeGroot, L. J. (Ed), New York: Grune & Stratton, pp. 1941–1962.

Stine, O. C, Hepenr, R., & Greenstreet, R. (1975). Correlation of blood pressure with skinfold thickness and protein levels. *Am. J. Dis. Child*, *129*, 905–911.

Stunkard, A. & Pestka. J. (1962). The physical activity of obese girls. *Am. J. Dis. Child*, *103*, 116–121.

Taylor, H. L., Jacobs, D. R., Schucker, B., Knudsen, J., Leon, A. S., & Debacker, G. (1978). A questionnaire for the assessment of leisure time physical activities. *J. Chron. Dis.*, *31*, 751–755.

United States Public Health Service, Division of Chronic Disease. (1966). *Obesity and Health: A Source Book of Current Information for Professional Health Personnel*. Washington, DC: U.S. Govt. Printing Office.

Van Itallie, T. B. (1977). Obesity: Prevalence and pathogenesis. In: *Diet Related to Killer Disease, II*. Hearings before select committee on nutrition and human need, United States Senate. Washington, DC: U.S. Govt. Printing Office, pp. 47–64.

Van Itallie, T. B. (1979). Obesity: Adverse effects on health and longevity. *Am. J. Clin. Nutr.*, *32*, 2723–2733.

Wallace, J. P., McKenzie T. L., & Nader, P. H. (1985). Observed vs. recalled exercise behavior: A validation of a seven day exercise recall for boys 11 to 13 years old. *Res. Qaurt.*, *56(2)*, 161–163.

Waxman, M., & Stunkard, A. J. (1980). Caloric intake and expenditure of obese boys. *J. Pediatr.*, *96(2)*, 187–193.

Weber, D. G., Kohl, H. W., Meredith, M. D., & Blair, S. N. (1986). An automated system for assessing physical fitness in school children. *Proceedings of the 1986 Public Health Conference on Records and Statistics*, National Center for Health Statistics: U.S. Govt. Printing Office: DHHS Publ. No. (PHS) 86–1214.

Wilkinson, P. W., Parkin, J. M., Pearlson, G., Strong, H., & Sykes, P. (1977). Energy intake and physical activity in obese children. *Br. Med. J.*, *756*.

Wilmore, J. H., Royce, J., Girandola, R. N., Katch, F. I., & Katch, V. L. (1970). Body composition changes with a 10-week program of jogging. *Med. Sci. Sports*, *2(3)*, 113–117.

Worsley, A., Coonan, W., Leitch, D., & Crawford, D. (1984). Slim and obese children's perceptions of physical activities. *Int. J. Ob.*, *8(3)*, 201–211.

Zack, P. M., Harlan, W. R., Leaverton, P. E., & Cornoni-Huntley, J. (1979). A longitudinal study of body fatness in childhood and adolescence. *J. Pediatr.*, *95(1)*, 126–130.

9

School-based Programs to Prevent or Reduce Obesity

GUY S. PARCEL, LAWRENCE W. GREEN, BARBARA A. BETTES
Center for Health Promotion Research and Development
The University of Texas Health Science Center at Houston
Houston, Texas

I. Introduction

The etiology of adult obesity appears to be centered as much in genetics and early childhood experiences with food and exercise as in adult behavior (Charney, Goodman, McBride, Lyon and Pratt, 1976; Brownell and Stunkard, 1980; Stunkard, et al., 1986). There is evidence that impending or actual obesity begins at ages six to nine years (Shapiro, et al., 1984), and that increases in obesity in this age range and through age 17 are associated with increases in levels of serum total cholesterol, serum triglycerides, and low-density lipoprotein cholesterol (Freedman, et al., 1985; Tokunaga, et al., 1982).

This chapter assesses the experience to date in designing and implementing experiments and programs to prevent or reduce obesity in school-aged children. A core feature of the argument that will be presented here is that school-based programs not only have the potential to provide a viable forum for interventions in childhood obesity, but they represent a valuable agency for reducing children's risk for adult obesity. More specifically, school-based programs can contribute to shifting social norms for exercise behavior (increasing energy expenditure) and for the eating behavior of children to reduce the excessive intake of simple sugars (candy, etc.), and high-fat foods, and increase consumption of complex carbohydrates (fruits, vegetables, etc.).

Concern with the prevention of children's *risk* for obesity, in addition to interventions for children who are already obese, arises from observations such as those of Frank, Webber, and Berenson (1982), who determined that the major source of energy for ten-year-olds was obtained from in-between meal eating (snacking). Combined with longitudinal data that indicate that obese children have a high probability of becoming obese adults (Charney, et al., 1976), such findings lead inevitably to the search for early interventions that will modify children's behavior and environment to reduce their risk for obesity. Schools seem an obvious place for interventions because of the potential for reaching large numbers of children and efficiently providing programs for risk reduction.

In the pages that follow, the discussion will focus first on components of obesity interventions in general that have been found to be effective. The next section reviews the studies that have been conducted to evaluate the effectiveness of school-based interventions to reduce or control weight in children or adolescents who are overweight or obese. The final section of the chapter summarizes major findings from past studies into a series of guidelines for policy and further research and presents a conceptualization for considering multiple influencing factors within a school-based intervention.

II. Research on Obesity Interventions

Coates and Thoreson (1978) reviewed the research on interventions for obesity in children and adolescents. They conclude that, in spite of some promising short-term results achieved with various types of interventions, clinically significant weight loss is rare, and when weight loss does occur, it is seldom maintained. While Coates and Thoreson acknowledge the possibility that obesity may be biogenetically determined in some individuals, they also argue that the negative results of the intervention studies reviewed were attributable to deficiencies in the intervention strategies employed by program designers and researchers. Among the less successful forms of intervention, they cite low calorie diets prescribed by others for the subjects, anorectic drugs, and other interventions which do not involve long-term changes in attitudes and behaviors.

Since this review, a number of intervention studies have produced more promising results using multi-component behavior modification approaches within clinical programs (e.g., Epstein, Wing, Steranchak, Dickson, and Michelson, 1980; Epstein, Wing, Koeske, Andrasi, and Ossip, 1981; Coates and Thoreson, 1981). A general conclusion arising from this and other research (e.g., Kirschenbaum, Harris, and Tomarken, 1984), is that involvement of parents and family as active participants in the intervention is a crucial determinant of success in long-term maintenance of weight loss. Kirschenbaum et al. (1984), for example, found that parental attendance in treatment sessions for their children facilitated maintenance of weight loss for both members of the dyad, and that correlations of weight loss for parent and child across the first year posttreatment were positive.

A second general conclusion is that interventions involving life-style changes in the area of physical activity have a greater likelihood of success, especially when coupled with behavior management techniques, such as contracting, modeling, and social reinforcement, than do interventions involving short-term changes in activity level (Epstein, Wing, Koeske, and Valoski, 1984). More importantly, there is substantial evidence for the importance of exercise in weight control for children and adolescents. Cohen, Gelfand, Dodd, Jensen, and Turner (1980), in a correlational study, found that children's continued participation in physical exercise, after termination of the intervention, was associated with the maintenance of weight loss found in this study in overweight children and adolescents. Cohen et al. (1980) suggest that participation in physical activity should be viewed as a self-regulation behavior, and that the maintenance of weight loss resulted from an enhancement of these children's ability to self-regulate. In support of this contention, they provide evidence that the parents of those children who had regained lost weight were involved in monitoring and regulating the child's diet, rather than the child's taking responsibility for his or her own diet.

Characteristics of the physical activity component may impact upon the effectiveness of an intervention. A series of studies by Epstein and his colleagues (Epstein, Wing, Koeske, Ossip and Beck, 1982; Epstein et al., 1984; Epstein et al., 1985), provide results from clinic-based studies that indicate that exposure to an exercise program is a predictor of maintenance of nonobesity; further, that diet plus exercise results in greater weight loss than diet alone; and, finally, that lifestyle exercise is more effective than programmed exercise for long-term weight maintenance. The authors suggest that this final result arose from a better adherence to lifestyle exercise changes (e.g., walking instead of riding, taking stairs instead of elevators, increasing walking, etc.), than for programmed, aerobic-type exercise.

An unfortunate aspect of this research, however, is that the programs reported are small-scale interventions for children who have been self-referred for treatment by parents. Thus, a substantial number of children may never have the opportunity to benefit from an intervention, since they may never be referred for one. Further, such programs may provide prohibitively expensive models for intervention on a larger scale. This is

Table I
School-based intervention studies for child or adolescent obesity

Study	Subjects	Intervention	Design	Follow-Up	Major Findings
Botvin, et al., 1979	n = 50 n = 69 7–8 grades 44% boys	NE PA BM (10 weeks)	Random Assignment of 4 *schools* To T or C	None	Significant Decrease in # of overweight students in experimental group; virtually no change in control group.
Brownell & Kaye, 1982	T: n = 63 C: n = 14 37 boys 40 girls 5–12 yrs.	NE PA BM (10 weeks)	Self-selection (Parental Permission) (Control group = 5 refusers & 9 randomly selected from another school)	None	T: 95.2% lost weight (X = −4.4 kg) C: 21.4% lost weight (X = +1.2 kg)
Collipp, 1975	n = 25 4th–6th grade	Phase I (6 weeks): PA Phase II (6 weeks): PA + Diet	One group	None	Phase I: no effect Phase II: Weight loss (X = 10 lbs.)
Foster, et al., 1985	T: n = 48 (50% boys) C: n = 41 Grades 2–5	PA + BM (12 weeks)	2 schools: T assigned to one C to other	18 weeks	*Posttreatment* T: decreased % overweight X = 5.3% Lost X = .15 kg C: increased % overweight X = 3% gained X 1.3 kg *Follow-Up* T: increased % overweight X = 1.7% gained X = 2.3 kg. C: decreased % overweight .5% gained X = 1.2 kg. (Parental involvement component had no effect)

Study	Sample	Intervention	Assignment	Follow-up	Results
Lansky & Brownell, 1982	boys n = 32 girls n = 39 aged 12–15	BM or PA + NE (15 weeks)	Random to classes in 3 schools. no untreated control	None	64% of B & 63% of PA + NE reduced % over ideal weight
Lansky & Vance 1983	T: n = 30 NT: n = 25 C: n = 59 45% boys 12–14 yrs.	T: RM & PA weighed @3 weeks NT: weighed pre 6 post (12 weeks) C: weighed	Random assignment to T/NT	None	T: Decreased % Overweight X = 5.71% NT: Decreased % Overweight X = 2.41 C: Decreased % Overweight X = 1.48% (Parental participation associated with weight Loss in T)
Ruppenthal & Gibbs, 1979	T: N = 14 boys 4/14 C: N = 28 boys 13/28 age: 5–10	T: PA & NE C: NE (5 months)	Self selected (Parent's Permission)	None	T: 13/14 decreased % overweight C: 3/28 decreased % overweight
Seltzer & Meyer 1970	T: N = 189 C: N = 161 ages 8–15	T: PA & NE C: Nothing (5–6 months)	Self selected (Chose to participate)	None	Measure: Ponderal Index Treatment / Control Elem Sch boys 81.3% improved vs 52.6% Elem Sch girls 70% improved vs 62.9% J.H.S. girls 58% improved vs 46.4%
Zakus et al. 1981	All girls age X = 14 yrs. T: N = 10 C: N = 12	NE + PA + BM (9 weeks)	Self selected (Chose to participate) one school	6 & 10 Months	At 10 month follow-up: T: decreased % OW X = 9.26% C: decreased % OW X = .86% (Nonsignificant differences at 3 & 6 months)

Notes: RM = Behavior Management
PA = Physical Activity
NE = Nutrition Education
T = Treatment Group
NT = No Treatment Group
C = Control Group

Criterion for inclusion in all studies: 10% over ideal bodyweight for age, height, & sex.

an important issue in view of our stated goal of the reduction of risk for adult obesity among children. As noted in the introduction, schools provide an attractive option for large-scale interventions since schools provide a larger and more continuous captive audience of children than any other context (Collipp, 1975).

III. School-based Interventions

In the past five years, there has been a concerted effort to design and implement school-based programs to treat obesity among school children. These efforts have met with some success and provide suggestive evidence for what constitutes a potentially successful intervention, although most do not provide long-term follow-ups. As can be seen in Table 1, programs that have an effect on weight loss tend to combine at least two of the three components (behavior management, nutrition education, and physical activity). There is also some indication that interventions with younger children are more successful than those with adolescents. Of the two studies that provide follow-up results (Foster, et al., 1985 and Zakus, et al., 1981), in only the Zakus et al., study did children maintain weight loss after termination of the program. It is notable that this study combined all three components, while the Foster et al. (1985), study included only physical activity and behavior management.

Among the most distinguishable features in programs directed at obesity in the context of the school is the degree to which they treat the energy intake and energy expenditure variables singly or in combination. Brownell and Stunkard (1980) demonstrated that the high correlation between these two energy balance variables and obesity in adults does not hold so consistently for children. That is, obese children appear to engage in as much physical activity as their normal-weight peers. Nevertheless, school-based programs that combine the two components of diet and exercise yield more promising results (e.g., Botvin, Cantlon, Carter, and Williams, 1979; Brownell and Kaye, 1982; Ruppental, and Gibbs, 1979; Zakus, et al 1981; Lansky and Brownell, 1982; Nelson, Catchings, and Pendleton, 1983; Collipp, 1975), than do programs concentrating more exclusively on eating behavior (Domke, Lando, and Robinson, 1981; Cosper, 1977). Collipp (1975), for example, found no change in weight for 25 children during a six-week period during which they exercised daily for one hour, but the same children experienced an average weight loss of ten pounds during a second six-weeks, in which exercise was combined with dietary prescriptions.

In addition, Brownell and Kaye (1982) demonstrated that behavior modification approaches can be combined with nutrition education and physical activity in a school-based programs to produce significant weight losses in obese children. It is noteworthy, in view of the family literature discussed earlier, that their program provided education for both the children and others in the children's social network (e.g., parents, teachers, physical education instructor, food service personnel, school administrators and the nurse's aide). Brownell and Kaye conclude that the social support provided by the involvement of others in the children's social networks was a significant factor in the overall success of their program. It is also noteworthy that nonobese children requested to join the intervention program, as well as obese children. This suggests that, not only can school- and family-based programs consist of similar components, they need also not be restricted to children targeted for obesity.

Further, the results of school-based studies indicate that similar issues are operative in both contexts. One of these issues relates to the degree to which physical activity components of the intervention result in increased physical activity in general; that is, whether or not life-style changes in physical activity occur, as opposed to program-specific increases in activity. Studies evaluating physical education programs in the United States have focused on measuring types of fitness, (i.e., strength, flexibility, and endurance), rather than changes in the proportion of body fat, or other physiological measures, in children who participate in such programs. A series of studies in Adelaide, Australia, have demonstrated that a long-term, daily exercise program at school which includes a minimum of twenty minutes of intensive physical activity can produce a significant reduction in body fat of elementary school children (Dwyer, Coonan, Worsley, and Leitch, 1979; Dwyer, Coonan, Leitch, Hetzel, and Baghurst, 1983). In a cross-sectional study, these investigators compared a group of ten-year olds who participated in a two-year program of intensive physical activity at school to a group who had regular physical education that emphasized skill training. The results revealed a significant difference in the percentage of children considered overweight, with 20.8% for the intensive physical activity group and 30.2% for the skill training group (Hetzel et al., 1983). Thus, a key factor in the effectiveness of school-based exercise programs in increasing energy expenditure is the ability of the programs to require and maintain participation and adherence in physical activity.

Another characteristic that has been associated with program success is the age group to which the intervention is geared. Programs aimed at younger (elementary school) children appear to have achieved better weight control results than those with junior high, adolescent and college-age youth (Seltzer and Mayer, 1970; Domke et al., 1981). This is not

surprising, in view of the fact that the degree to which a program suc-
ceeds in bringing about life-style changes is strongly related to the success
of an intervention. Clearly, health-related habits become more intran-
sigent as a child matures, and are more malleable in preschool and
elementary school children than in adolescents.

A third feature that has been found to influence the success of school-
based programs is the degree to which parents are involved, and the type
of involvement. Parental involvement with the program produces better
results than programs without, and degree of parental involvement within
programs correlates with amount of weight loss (Lansky and Vance, 1983;
Brownell and Kaye, 1982; Nelson et al., 1985). Further, programs that
simply instruct parents in nutritional guidelines and diet planning are less
successful that those that aid parents in enabling the child to modify his or
her behavior.

Table 1 provides a summary of the school-based interventions to control
weight for obese children and adolescents. These studies collectively
provide evidence that successful programs for weight control in children
require combinations of intervention strategies, and that a single intervention approach is unlikely to be effective.

IV. Future Direction for Research and Programs

A strong heuristic case, in addition to the empirical evidence just cited,
can be made for using schools as a major delivery system for programs to
prevent or reduce childhood obesity. The schools provide easy access to
children, continuous and concentrated contact can be maintained, programs
can be made more cost effective, and intervention can take place within
the context of the child's natural environment. There is evidence that
school-based programs can be effective in accomplishing improved weight
control in children. However, a number of issues have not been addressed,
and more investigative work is needed to define more clearly the school's
role.

A. Reducing risk for the population of school children

It has been argued that a major weakness of clinic-based intervention
research is the focus on children who have been identified as obese and
who have been referred for treatment for obesity. A similar criticism can
be made of school-based programs. That is, most of these studies have
focused on interventions for children who are identified by the researchers
or the school nurse as obese. Further, the goal has been either to reduce

weight or to slow down the rate of weight gain. Little attention has been paid to a population-based approach which would use the schools to attempt to reduce the number of children who become obese, or to modify behavioral and environmental conditions which might be contributory to maintaining obesity in children. Three components of the school program itself can be identified as having potential for contributing to the prevention of obesity: the physical education program, classroom health education, and the school food service.

The Adelaide studies have important implications for examining the role of school physical education programs in the United States. In the Adelaide studies (Dwyer et al., 1983), the physical activity program included all children in the school, rather than children identified as obese or at-risk. Nevertheless, the fitness program had a significant impact, not only on the condition of the "average" child, but also on the condition of those at the upper end of the distribution.

Physical education programs in elementary schools continue to place a primary emphasis on skill training and organized games and sports, with very little time devoted to intensive or aerobic types of activities. For example, in an observational study of diet and exercise behavior in elementary school children (Parcel et al., 1987), observations of children in physical education classes revealed that an average of less than three minutes out of a 40-minute physical education class was spent in vigorous activity. The remainder of the time was spent on organization, attendance-taking, and so on. Yet, given the opportunity, children will engage in fitness-oriented activities. In this same study, left on their own at recess, children spent over 70% of their time moving. Physical education classes in elementary schools could be a major resource for increasing the energy expenditure of young children. Involvement of overweight children in vigorous activity in physical education classes throughout the five or six years of elementary school could contribute not only to increased energy expenditure, but to developing an expectation for being active and creating a social norm for frequent and regular physical activity.

Possible areas for future investigations include a determination of the feasibility of school physical education programs' shifting the emphasis from skill training and sports to maintaining moderate to vigorous physical activity. Research will be needed to document the longitudinal effects of physical education programs which emphasize intensive activity on percent body fat and the prevalence of obesity.

With regard to classroom health education, heart healthy school health education programs that take a behavioral approach to reducing cardiovascular disease risk factors have been developed and field tested (Coates, Jeffrey, and Slinkard, 1981; Perry, Mullis, and Maile, 1985; Parcel et al.,

1987). Additional research is needed to determine the contribution these types of health education interventions can make in assisting children in making effective decisions and in modifying eating and exercise behavior related to weight control. It is clear that successful classroom interventions incorporate some of the basic principles of behavior management and social learning theory into the program. In the Adelaide studies, for example, one of the interventions included self-monitoring and the teaching of techniques for behavior change. Children in the self-monitoring group showed a greater reduction in skinfold measurements and greater improved performance in some of the fitness measures as compared to other groups who participated in the same intensive physical education program but did not include self-monitoring (Hetzel et al., 1983). These results are related to those of Cohen et al. (1980) who proposed that the mechanism of change in their study was not physical activity per se, but enhancement of the ability to control one's own behavior eventuated by the exercise intervention.

Thus, it can be argued that many of the skills affected by school-based programs are closely related to success in other school-related activities, and school health education programs could be used not only to teach children the content related to physical activity and nutrition, but also to teach children how to monitor diet and exercise behavior, how to set goals for changes, and techniques for initiating and maintaining behavior change.

In combination with major changes in the schools' physical education program and classroom health education, attention should also focus on how the school environment itself can be changed to support diet and exercise changes. For example, the efficacy of nutrition interventions is severely limited by the availability of high-fat, high-calorie foods in the school cafeteria. Since the majority of calories consumed by children come from snacks (Frank et al., 1982), a primary target of nutrition education for elementary school children should be snack-type food, to shift both the type and amount of food consumed to reduce excessive sugar, fat, and sodium intake. In addition, the food served in the school cafeteria should conform with dietary goals for reduced fat, sodium and sugar (Parcel et al., 1987). School snack bars, vending machines, and other food programs should all be examined to ensure that children are getting consistent messages about healthy food and appropriate eating behavior. Further research is needed to determine if changes made in school food service programs will have a significant impact on children's daily food consumption and whether practices learned and reinforced in the school program will generalize to out-of-school behavior.

Schools do not approach health interventions on a categorical basis.

Therefore, the avenues of investigation that have been suggested here will need to be placed within a broader context than prevention of obesity. It has been suggested that school health promotion programs can incorporate all of the necessary components of effective interventions in the context of promoting health for the purpose of improving performance in schools and reducing risk factors for chronic disease (Green, 1985; Kolbe et al., 1986). Of interest in the prevention of childhood obesity is the question of whether or not the effects of health intervention programs generalize to other health behaviors. That is, can health promotion programs that target a specific problem (e.g., obesity), through creating an environment favorable to enabling and reinforcing behavior change, also have an impact upon the prevalence of other health problems among school children?

B. Programs for children at greatest risk

The school's role in providing interventions for children who are obese or at risk for obesity remains poorly defined. Although a number of interventions have shown promising results for short-term weight control, it is not known if short-term results will be maintained through adolescence and into adulthood. It is also unclear as to the likelihood that school administrators will see interventions for obese children as a responsibility of the educational system and therefore be willing to allocate resources for special programs. Thus, in addition to the specific short-term questions requiring further investigation, there is a need for longitudinal studies to determine the types of programs needed to maintain weight control, and for dissemination and diffusion studies to develop and evaluate methods for implementing effective programs outside of experimental situations.

The intractability of obesity throughout the lifespan argues convincingly for early and multifaceted interventions that encompass multiple contexts of children's lives. The most successful interventions in Table 1 are those that successfully merged the many different relationships children have with others into a unified project. Investigations should continue to examine the additive effects of intervening with parents and other key adults within the obese child's environment. The school nurse could serve as a central figure to coordinate programs in the school with the child's family and health care providers. The school nurse may be the key professional in the schools to enable a generalization of programs demonstrated to be effective under experimental conditions. School-based programs for obese children should also be concerned with the potential harmful effects of interventions. Research in this area should include an assessment of such issues as labeling, coercion and excessive food restrictions (Mallick, 1983)

V. Summary of Current Knowledge

There is evidence to suggest that schools have the potential of contributing to both the prevention and the treatment of childhood obesity. The specific role that schools should take is not well defined and is difficult to determine with current data. We need to know more about the long-term effects of school-based interventions for obese children and the contribution that can be made by schoool health promotion programs that include behavioral change strategies and environmental support. As with other health-related problems affecting children and youth, schools cannot be viewed as the only source for solutions. The school's role in preventing and treating childhood obesity must be consistent with the goals and responsibilities of the educational system, and be conceptualized as only one part of broader community and health care system interventions.

Specific guidelines for policy and further research that would seem to be suggested by the results of studies discussed in this review include the following:

1. Interventions should include components directed both at food intake and at energy expenditure.
2. The dietary component of interventions should provide for parental involvement and for behavior modification and environmental modification.
3. The energy expenditure component should emphasize continuous, vigorous exercise rather than short-burst competitive activities characteristic of many physical education programs in schools. For overweight children, changes in lifestyle exercise should be used to increase energy expenditures and self-management skills.
4. Food service personnel and food purchasing and preparation policies for schools require attention in any comprehensive program directed at obesity control in schools.
5. For both diet and exercise components of school-based obesity control programs, self-monitoring appears to be an important skill to be developed in the child, probably for reasons of reinforcement and feedback in the learning process.
6. Involvement of peers in the education of individual children and adolescents appears to be helpful in building a supportive social climate and norm for the dietary or exercise behavior.

Finally, an issue that must be examined is whether intervention programs specific to *obesity* are necessary, or whether a more general approach, aimed at improving children's health and health-related behaviors starting with entry into schools, would be effective not only in preventing obesity in later childhood and adolescence, but also in treating cases of obesity within the school population. As Coates & Thoreson (1978) argue, the factors that influence obesity are learned and maintained early in life at the level of the family and the culture. Hence, the most successful form of intervention would be early prevention which includes members of the child's family as well as representative members of the society as a whole.

In summary, it has been argued that the success of obesity interventions is contingent upon the degree to which the intervention incorporates a variety of individuals in the child's environment, as well as all the contexts in which the child functions into the intervention. Programs that focus only on one component, such as adding an extra physical education class, cannot be as successful as those that promote behaviors and attitudes which are reflected in physical activity and other self-regulating behaviors. Peer and parent involvement is also important, and the degree to which teachers and other school personnel can be involved serves to increase the program's likelihood of success.

References

Botvin, G. J., Cantlon, A., Carter, B. J., & Williams, C. L. (1979). Reducing adolescent obesity through a school health program. *Journal of Pediatrics, 86* (6), 1060–1062.

Brownell, K. D., & Kaye, F. S. (1982). A school-based behavior modification, nutrition education, and physical activity program for obese children. *American Journal of Clinical Nutrition, 35,* 277–283.

Brownell, K. D., & Stunkard, A. J. (1980). Physical activity in the development and control of obesity. In A. J. Stunkard (ed.), *Obesity,* Philadelphia: Saunders.

Charney, E., Goodman, H. C., McBride, M., Lyon, B., & Pratt, B. (1976). Childhood antecedents of adult obesity: Do chubby infants become obese adults? *New England Journal of Medicine, 295,* 6–9.

Coates, T. J., & Thoreson, C. E. (1978). Treating obesity in children and adolescents: A review. *American Journal of Public Health, 68(2),* 143–151.

Coates, T. J., & Thoreson, C. E. (1981). The efficacy of a multicomponent self-control program in modifying the eating habits and weight of three obese adolescents. *Behavior Therapy, 12,* 383–399.

Coates T. J., Jeffrey R. W., & Slinkard, L. A. (1981). Heart healthy eating and exercise: Introducing and maintaining changes in health behaviors. *American Journal of Public Health 71,* 15–23.

Cohen, E. A., Gelfand, D. M., Dodd, D. K., Jensen, J., & Turner, C. (1980). Self-control practices associated with weight loss maintenance in children and adolescents. *Behavior Therapy, 11,* 26–37.

Collipp, P. J. (May, 1975). An obesity program in public schools. *Pediatric Annals,* 276–282.

Cosper, B. A., Hayslip, D. E., & Foree, S. B. (1977). The effect of nutrition education on dietary habits of fifth graders. *Journal of School Health, 47* (8), 475–477.

Domke, J. A., Lando, H. A., & Robinson, D. C. (1981). A behavioral weight control program for residence hall students. *Journal of Counseling Psychology, 28* (4), 365–368.

Dwyer, T., Coonan, W. E., Leitch, D. R., Hetzel, B. S., & Baghurst, P. A. (1983). An investigation of the effects of daily physical activity on the health of primary school students in South Australia. *International Journal of Epidemiology, 121* (3), 308–313.

Dwyer, T., Coonan, W. E., Worsley, A., & Leitch, D. R. (1979). An assessment of the effects of two physical activity programs on coronary heart disease risk factors in primary school children. *Community Health Studies, 3,* 196–202.

Epstein, L. H., Wing, R. R., Koeske, R., Andrasi, K. F., & Ossip, D. J. (1981). Child and parent weight loss in family-based behavior modification programs. *Journal of Consulting and Clinical Psychology, 49,* 674–686.

Epstein, L. H., Wing, R. R., Koeske, R., Ossip, D., & Beck, S. (1982). A comparison of life-style changes and programmed aerobic exercise on weight and fitness changes in obese children. *Behavior Therapy, 13,* 651–665.

Epstein, L. H., Wing, R. R., Koeske, R., & Valoski, A., (1984). Effects of diet plus exercise on weight change in parents and children. *Journal of Consulting and Clinical Psychology, 52(3),* 429–437.

Epstein, L. H., Wing., R. R., Penner, B. C., & Kress, M. J. (1985). Effect of diet and controlled exercise on weight loss in obese children. *Journal of Pediatrics, 107,* 358–361.

Epstein, L. H., Wing, R. R., Steranchak, L., Dickson, B., & Michelson, J. (1980). Comparison of family-based behavior modification and nutrition for childhood obesity. *Journal of Pediatric Psychology, 5,* 23–36.

Foster, G. D., Wadden, T. A., Brownell, K. D. (1985). Peer-led program for the treatment and prevention of obesity in the schools. *Journal of Consulting and Clinical Psychology, 53,* 538–540.

Frank, G. C., Webber, L. S., & Berenson, G. S. (1982). Dietary studies of infants and children: The Bogalusa Heart Study. In T. J. Coates, A. C. Petersen, & C. Perry (eds.), *Promoting Adolescent Health,* New York: Academic Press.

Freedman, B. S., Burke, G. L., Harsha, D. W., Srinivasan, S. R., Cresenta, J. L., Webber, L. S., & Berenson, G. S. (1985). Relationship of changes in obesity to serum lipid and lipoprotein changes in childhood and adolescence. *Journal of the American Medical Association 254* (4), 515–520.

Green, L. W. (1985). Some challenges to health services research on children and the elderly. *Health Services Research 19,* 793–815.

Hetzel, B. S., Worsley, A., Maynard, E. J., Baghurst, P. A., Coonan, W., & Dwyer, T. (November, 1983). *Reduction of CHD risk factors by integrated school based physical health education programs in Australian 10-year-old children.* Paper presented at the World Health Organization, Meeting of Investigators on Epidemiological Studies of Atherosclerosis Precursors in Children, Geneva.

Kirschenbaum, D. S., Harris, E. S., & Tomarken, A. J. (1984). Effects of parental involvement in behavioral weight loss therapy for preadolescents. *Behavior Therapy, 15,* 485–500.

Kolbe, L. J., Green, L. W., Foreyt, J., Darnell, L., Goodrick, K., Williams, H., Ward, D., Korton, A. S., Karacan, I., Widmeyer, R., & Stainbrook, G. (1986). Appropriate functions of health education in schools: Improving health and cognitive performance. In N. Krasnegor, J. Arasteh, & M. Cataldo, (Eds.), *Child Health Behavior: A Behavioral Pediatrics Perspective.* New York: John Wiley and Sons.

Lansky, D., & Brownell, K. D. (1982). Composition of School-based treatments of adolescent obesity *Journal of School Health, 52,* 384–387.

Lansky, D., & Vance, M. A. (1983). School-based intervention for adolescent obesity:

Analysis of treatment, randomly selected control and self-selected control subjects. *Journal of Consulting and Clinical Psychology, 51* (1), 147–148.

Mallick, M. J. (1983). Health hazards of obesity and weight control in children: A review of the literature. *American Journal of Public Health 73* (1), 78–82.

Nelson, E. C., Catchings, M. W., & Pendleton, T. B. (1983). Weight reduction and maintenance for overweight, mentally retarded students, ages 9–17. *Journal of School Health, 53* (6) 380–381.

Parcel, G. S., Simons-Morton, B., O'Hara, N., Baranowski, T., Kolbe, L., & Bee, D. (1987). School promotion of healthful diet and exercise behavior: An integration of organizational change and social learning theory interventions. *Journal of School Health, 57* (4) 150–156.

Perry, C. L., Mullis, R. M., & Maile, M. C. (1985). Modifying the eating behavior of young children. *Journal of School Health, 55* (10), 399–402.

Ruppenthal, B., & Gibbs, E. (1979). Treating childhood obesity in a public school setting. *Journal of School Health, 49 (10),* 569–571.

Seltzer, C. C., & Mayer, J. (1970). An effective weight control program in a public school system. *American Journal of Public Health, 60* (4), 679–689.

Shapiro, L. R., Crawford, P. B., Clark, M. J., Pearson, D. L., Raz, J., & Huenemann, R. L. (1984). Obesity prognosis: A longitudinal study of children from the age of 6 months to 9 years. *American Journal of Public Health, 74* (9), 968–972.

Stunkard, A. J., Sorensen, T. I., Hanis, C., Teasdale, T. W., Chakraborty, R., Schull, W. J., & Schulsinger, F. (1986). An adoption study of human obesity. *New England Journal of Medicine, 314* (4), 193–198.

Tokunaga, K., Ishikawa, K., Sudo, H., Matsuzawa, Y., Yamamoto, A., & Tarui, S. (1982). Serum lipoprotein profile in Japanese obese children. *International Journal of Obesity, 6,* 399–404.

Van Biervliet, J. P., & DeWijn, J. F. (1981). Blood lipid values in obese children. *Acta Paediatrica Belgica, 31,* 27–34.

Williams, C. L. (1981). Prevention and treatment of childhood obesity in a public school setting. *Pediatric Annals, 13* (6), 482–483, 486–487, 490.

Zakus, G., Chin, M. L., Cooper, H., Makovsky, E., & Merrill, C. (1981). Treating adolescent obesity: A pilot project in a school. *Journal of School Health,* December, 663–666.

IV

TREATMENT

10

Approaches to the Clinical Evaluation of Obesity in Children

SUE Y.S. KIMM
School of Medicine
University of Pittsburgh
Pittsburgh, Pennsylvania

I. Introduction

Childhood obesity is a difficult condition to treat in the usual clinical setting. At present, there is no consensus among medical professionals as to whom to treat, what levels and types of intervention to use, and what kind of clinical evaluation would be appropriate in treating an obese child. Because of so much uncertainty surrounding childhood obesity, the physician and the obese pediatric patient as well as his/her parents are frequently prevented from taking more active roles.

The purpose of this chapter is to discuss those areas of clinical evaluation which would offer rational and practical approaches to the clinical management of childhood obesity. This paper outlines specific issues and suggestions related to medical evaluation, psychosocial assessment, surveillance of clinical progress, and safety monitoring for the potentially adverse effects of dietary restrictions in growing children.

II. Medical Evaluation

The initial medical evaluation of an obese child should include a search for the causes of obesity in that child. It should also assess the health and psychosocial consequences of the child's obesity.

161

A.   Searching for Causes of Obesity

When a physician sees a child with moderate to severe obesity, there is always the question of whether it might be primary or secondary obesity, the latter being due to an underlying endocrine disorder. The perennial question from parents concerning an obese child is whether or not there is an underlying hormonal disorder. A commonly heard statement is, "Doctor, my child really does not eat that much. I think it's his/her glands." Thyroid function tests are often carried out to address this question and, in most instances, they suggest normal thyroid function. Tests for adrenal dysfunction are usually similarly negative. As third party payment systems generally do not underwrite obesity-related medical costs, laboratory evaluation should be kept to the basic minimum commensurate with good clinical practice. Diagnostic laboratory tests should be carried out for clinical indications other than excessive body weight.

As in most clinical situations, the first and most useful diagnostic tool is that of careful medical history-taking. Although the majority of obese children have exogenous obesity, there are rare congenital types of obesity such as Prader-Willi or Laurence-Moon-Biedl syndromes, and Alstrom's disease, which often have typical histories and clinical features. There are no laboratory tests specifically diagnostic for these conditions, but they can be ruled out by historical information and physical examination. Chromosomal abnormalities have been associated with Prader-Willi syndrome, but not in all cases; consequently, cytogenetic studies are not very helpful in the typical clinical evaluation of a child suspected of having this disorder.

When it comes to potential endocrine causes of obesity, the best initial diagnostic tool is a growth chart. In general, children with primary obesity have either normal or accelerated linear growth. In ten years of clinical experience at the Duke Pediatric Obesity Clinic, the mean relative height (actual height divided by the fiftieth percentile height for age, multiplied by 100) of our 332 obese subjects was above 100%. It is not at all uncommon to see an obese child's height in the 90th, or greater than the 95th percentile line on the growth chart. The exact opposite trend is seen in hypothyroidism and Cushing's disease, both of which are associated with obesity. As such endocrine disorders become symptomatic, these clinical entities manifest as obesity as well as short stature since there is a concomitant deceleration of linear growth. Therefore, if normal or accelerated linear growth is seen, one can reasonably assume that the child has exogenous or primary obesity, and further laboratory tests to rule out endocrine disease are not warranted.

B. Assessing the Consequences of Obesity

A proper medical evaluation of obesity should include investigation of morbidity associated with obesity. Obesity has been associated with elevated blood pressure, less favorable plasma lipid profiles, hyperglycemia, hyperinsulinemia, hypoventilation syndrome, and sleep apnea. The association between obesity, mortality, and such coronary heart disease (CHD) risk factors as hypertension or unfavorable plasma lipid patterns is better established in adults (Foster and Burton, 1985; Van Itallie, 1985; Garrison and Castelli, 1985; Bjorntorp, 1985; Messerli, 1982; Lucas et al., 1985). However, study of healthy male adolescents with low-moderate to moderate physical fitness revealed a positive association between body mass index (BMI), systolic and diastolic blood pressure readings, and plasma triglyceride levels, and revealed a negative association between BMI and level of plasma high density lipoprotein cholesterol HDL-C and exercise duration (Fripp et al., 1985). Longitudinal studies from Bogalusa, Louisiana, and Muscatine, Iowa, have found that obese children who remain obese tended to also have persistence of higher blood lipids and higher blood pressure (Aristimuno et al., 1984, Lauer et al., 1984, Friedman et al., 1985 and Berenson et al., 1982). One of the characteristics of childhood obesity is that body weights of obese children over time tend to "track" along the same elevated growth curve (Johnston, 1985). Further, five-year follow-up of the Bogalusa cohort (mean age was 13.6 years at follow-up time) revealed that changes in triceps skinfold thickness were positively correlated with serum levels of total cholesterol, low density lipoprotein cholesterol (LDL-C), and triglycerides, and inversely associated with HDL-C (Friedman et al., 1985). There may also be increased orthopedic problems such as genu valgum and slipped capital femoral epiphysis with associated hip pain, conditions which sometimes require surgical repair (Dietz, 1983). In rare instances, Blount's disease (tibia vara) is also seen (Kelsey et al., 1972).

Less well-known conditions associated with obesity are gallbladder disease, hepatic steatosis, menstrual irregularities, trauma to the weight-bearing joints, increased hemoglobin concentration, and possibly immunologic impairment (Bray, 1985). However, these complications have been observed primarily in adult subjects. Severe or more morbid obesity has been associated with cardiopulmonary complications, such as Pickwickian syndrome, and cases have been observed in very obese children (Riley, Santiago and Edelman, 1976).

Although long-term effects are not generally viewed as immediate complications of childhood obesity, the following questions can be posed in reviewing the subject of complications of obesity in children. Childhood obesity is generally viewed as hypercellular as well as hypertrophic (Knittle, et al., 1979). This in turn may have implications for increasing the risk for adolescent and adult obesity. It has been reported that between 30 and 64% of the relative adiposity of an adolescent may be predicted by adiposity measured between ages six and 11 years (Zack et al., 1979 and Aarn, 1985). Obesity has been linked with increased risk for certain cancers including breast cancer (Garfinkel, 1985). However, these considerations are not immediately relevant to the clinical evaluation of an obese child.

Much has been written about the psychological factors related to obesity. It is assumed that obesity is associated with poor self-esteem (Wadden and Stunkard, 1985). Although a debate continues whether this is true for children, low self-concept measures can be a consequence of childhood obesity.

Finally, in the clinical setting, should there be any "routine" laboratory assessments for the consequences of obesity? Since elevated blood lipids are often a consequence of the life-style and dietary habits that have led to the child's current obesity, lipid determinations can be informative and of aid both in counseling the child and family and for follow-up. Blood lipid changes associated with obesity may include increases in total and LDL-C and triglyceride levels. At times, there may be a decrease in HDL-C levels. The initial lipid "profile" can serve as a useful means of monitoring clinical progress as the child continues with weight reduction. Further, when there is a family history of premature-onset CHD or hyperlipidemia, determination of the blood lipid profiles of accompanying family members would be informative and helpful for family counseling. Such testing can be a useful adjuvant for motivating the family to institute appropriate behavioral and dietary changes.

When elevated blood pressure is seen in an obese child, it needs to be assessed in the context of the family history, the child's body stature, and the actual blood pressure level. Data from the Bogalusa study indicate that elevated blood pressure in the obese child tends to remain elevated over time (Aristimuno et al., 1984). The Bogalusa study also revealed a close interrelationship between obesity and carbohydrate and insulin metabolism (Aristimuno et al., 1984 and Berenson et al., 1982). A linkage between obesity and elevation of levels of serum lipids and pre-beta and beta-lipoproteins, accompanied by hyperinsulinism, was noted even in those children with only mild obesity in the Bogalusa cohort. Thus, fasting blood glucose and/or urine glucose dipstick tests may be helpful as simple measures in uncovering Type II diabetes. It should be also noted that adolescent girls taking oral contraceptive agents may have a greater frequency of elevated blood pressure and lipid abnormalities associated with their obesity.

Those children with extreme degrees of obesity are also at high risk for potentially catastrophic sleep apnea. The physician should therefore take a careful history in the extremely obese child of increased somnolence, i.e., falling asleep in front of the TV, snoring, and enuresis associated with "deep" sleep (particularly in males). Pulmonary function studies should be undertaken to serve as part of the initial clinical assessment. In a series of 13 extremely obese children (aged 6–17 years with mean percent ideal body weight of 178) studied at the Duke Medical Center, the mean oxygen saturation of arterialized capillary blood gases was 78% (range 56–99%). One four-year-old male child had sleep apnea and was successfully resuscitated; he weighed 100 pounds at that age.

III. Psychosocial Evaluation

There are several levels of psychosocial evaluation which can be carried out in the usual clinical setting. At the first level, one can assess the way in which the child is referred to the clinic. Is this a self-referral or a referral by health professionals? There is currently a lack of consensus among pediatricians regarding the optimal treatment of childhood obesity, and there is also prevailing pessimism regarding the effectiveness of dietary therapy. Thus, not infrequently, the mother takes charge on her own by asking her friends and neighbors for referral information or by calling the nearest hospital. Self-referral can be assumed to indicate a high motivation level in the caretaker. In such an instance, the child will be more likely to be situated in a household milieu supportive of his treatment.

The nature of the chief complaint, as stated by the accompanying adult, gives an indication of the parental perception of the child's obesity. At the Duke Medical Center, we have (not infrequently) encountered mothers of obese children who state that they came to the clinic, not because they felt that their child was obese, but because they were requested either by their family physician or pediatrician to seek further care for the child's obesity. This is generally seen in family units where adult members are obese and thinness is not necessarily viewed as a desirable trait. Again, the formulation of the specific chief complaint serves as a gross indicator of the parents' level of concern and/or awareness regarding the child's obesity. It may signal whether or not the parents are more apt to play a passive or active role in any weight reduction-related activities.

Another important psychosocial assessment is the evaluation of the "ecological" setting for each child. This includes the overall family life-style such as food intake patterns, physical activity patterns, and the preferred family leisure activities. This ecological assessment should include the taking of a family history of obesity and of past and current attempts at weight reduction and the effectiveness of such efforts. Information is also sought regarding any overt eating disorders such as anorexia nervosa or bulimia among the family members. Ecological assessment should also include the nature and level of the parents' or caretaker's willingness to provide a supportive milieu for the child's weight reduction. This includes the willingness of the family to follow the same menu plan for the whole family (the distinction between diets of non-obese and obese members being the portion size), willingness to participate in weight reduction for themselves by allowing us to weigh them at each visit, their willingness to provide appropriate follow-up care by bringing the child for scheduled appointments, and their willingness to provide appropriate rewards for a contract goal for each clinic visit.

Psychological evaluation of the child in the usual primary care setting should be simple in order to be practicable. For instance, obtaining a clinical impression of the child's motivation toward weight reduction can serve as a helpful guide in predicting clinical outcome. One may approach this by asking the child if he/she is aware of the reason for this clinic visit and if he/she wishes to lose weight, and if so, why. We then ask for the child's perception of approaches to weight reduction. This can serve as a general indicator of the child's knowledge regarding dietary modification for weight reduction. Thus, by asking some simple questions, one can quickly ascertain the child's own perception of his/her current weight status, motivation for weight control, and knowledge of and attitude toward dietary restriction. This can aid in identifying potential barriers to effective therapy.

Unless there is an indication of a significant psychological disturbance, extensive psychological assessment in the usual primary care setting is neither warranted nor practical. If possible, however, there should be a routine and standardized way of assessing the child's self-concept, since obese children purportedly have disturbed self-images. The Piers-Harris test is a widely used scale with available normative standards and with field experience of its use in black children as well (Piers, 1969, Piers, 1977 and Wolf et al., 1982). At Duke, we have been administering the Piers-Harris questionnaire to assess self-concept measures in an obese childhood clinic population. At present, this is mainly for research purposes rather than for clinical reasons, but we are hopeful that when used properly, it could serve as a clinically useful tool for assessing the child's self-concept. With some modifications it might also be used for evaluating areas of possible psychological vulnerability in the obese child. The results of our analysis of Piers-Harris tests in 130 obese children reveal that there is considerable heterogeneity in self-concept measures among obese children. In general, girls and non-white children showed the lowest self-concept scores. Also, the areas of particularly low scores on the Piers-Harris subscales (Behavior, Intellectual and School Status, Physical Appearance and Attributes, Anxiety, Popularity, and Happiness and Satisfaction) are different for different gender, age, race, and relative-weight groups of obese children. At present there is no published information on the changes in measures of self-concept with weight loss in children. However, Piers-Harris scores have been shown to predict compliance with medication-taking for chronic disease in children (Litt, et al., 1982). Therefore, Piers-Harris scores may help in predicting successful outcomes for weight reduction. Further, those children with low scores on the Piers-Harris scale, would most likely need a more systematic psychological evaluation and further counseling. More research data are needed, however, before incorporating an instrument such as the Piers-Harris test as a "routine" clinical tool in the care of an obese child.

IV. Surveillance for Clinical Improvement

Proper evaluation during treatment must include a measure of the actual changes in adiposity such as changes in skinfold thickness, as growing children may become heavier in weight because of an increase in lean body mass while at the same time, they may be shedding fat which has lower density. If a skinfold caliper is not readily available, waist measurement may be a helpful measure in following changes in body habitus; this decrease in volume of adipose tissue may not be readily apparent if one were to follow body weights only.

An important part of clinical surveillance should include follow-up assessment of those clinical findings, be they blood pressure, blood lipids, glucose, or blood gases and/or pulmonary function tests which were abnormal at entry. Follow-up measurements in these areas are not only important in assessing clinical improvement but also are useful in providing positive reinforcement to help with patient motivation. There may be a "threshold" effect in the amount of adiposity lost before observing psychological, biochemical, and clinical improvement; however, for blood pressure and plasma triglycerides, modest weight reduction often brings significant improvement. Frequently, parents observe increased physical activity and improved exercise tolerance when the child loses weight. If possible, the impact of weight changes on the psychological status of the child should be reassessed. Qualitative measures which may be assessed are school performance and both the child's and parents' perception of the child's peer interactions. However, improvements may be due to the "placebo effect" of the extra attention asociated with treatment rather than to any actual weight loss.

As a regular follow-up measure, we also monitor the motivational levels of the child and accompanying family members. Frequently heard complaints which may denote waning motivation for dietary therapy are "becoming tired of the diet" or "being bored with it." Motivational levels can also improve with weight reduction. This is indicated when parents describe coping skills the child has acquired regarding eating at social gatherings or at school, or when parents note increasing participation by the child in food preparation and food serving.

The surveillance schema for monitoring clinical improvement should also include those family members who had abnormal blood pressure and/or blood lipid levels at entry. Weigh-in of the accompanying adult members is routinely done at the Duke Pediatric Obesity Clinic. Follow-up blood pressure and blood lipid measurements are carried out period-ically only in those family members with abnormal baseline measure-ments.

V. Safety Monitoring

An evaluation protocol which monitors the safety of treatment should be part of any obesity management program. Its aim is to detect potential adverse effects of dietary restriction in growing children. Again, as in the initial medical evaluation, the most clinically useful tools are dietary history and the growth chart. Dietary restriction should be targeted at calories only and not at other nutrients. If the child had been fasting or was on a bizarre restricted diet, then one needs to assess what potential nutrients might be lacking from such restricted dietary patterns. Often a careful dietary history can help indicate any need for further diagnostic evaluation for specific nutrient-associated clinical disorders. In general, traditional biochemical measures to assess protein nutriture, such as total serum protein and albumin, have insufficient sensitivity or specificity as a useful laboratory aid in diagnosing early mild protein undernutrition. In a young growing child, reasonable clinical evaluation may be the use of an estimate of lean body mass as mid-arm muscle area (MAMA in mm^2)

calculated from triceps skinfold thickness (TSF in mm) and mid-arm circumferences (MAC in mm) based on the formula,

$$MAMA = \frac{(MAC - \pi TSF)^2}{4\pi}$$

Although, normative standards for MAMA have been developed from population surveys, their ranges are wide (Frisancho, 1981). However, intraindividual variability can be minimal when measurements are carefully made. Thus, MAMA can be a useful clinical tool for safety monitoring of individual patients. Serial measures of MAMA can be particularly helpful in those fortunate instances of dramatic weight reduction over relatively short spans of time. In general, children with primary obesity tend to have higher values of MAMA; therefore, they tend to be overweight as well as obese (Forbes, 1964). Even with dramatic weight reduction, MAMA remains high when compared to age-and sex-adjusted population standards, but within the individual child MAMA usually remains unchanged over a period of several months, denoting no detectable decrease in body protein stores.

Recently, bioelectrical impedance measurements are becoming more widely used to estimate body fat as well as fat-free mass (Lukaski, et al., 1985). This method is safe, noninvasive, provides rapid measurements, and is relatively simple to use. However, normative standards have not yet been worked out for children, and validation of this method will be needed in subjects with abnormal body composition such as very obese children. Growth and growth velocity charts are still the best and most readily available clinical tools for safety monitoring since the overall health of the child is best reflected in normal growth patterns. A child should maintain his or her rate of linear growth even in the face of dramatic weight loss. If the rate of linear growth trails off, one should first assess the child's stage of puberty and ascertain whether or not the child has experienced pubescence. In general, obese children mature earlier than do their normal-weight counterparts. For instance, a Fels Institute study noted that children who were fatter at 8.5−9.5 years reached menarche and tibial union earlier than their leaner counterparts (Garn and Haskell, 1960). The extremes of fatness were characterized by marked differences in rates of growth and up to 5 years' difference in menarcheal age. A study reported by Dietz noted deceleration of height growth velocity with weight reduction (Dietz and Hartung, 1985). Preliminary findings from our study at Duke indicate that there may be a slight deceleration in height velocity. However, in our cohort, these patients, along with their marked degree of obesity, also had markedly accelerated linear growth. As their weights became more "normalized," so, too, did their heights, which had been outliers on their growth charts, i.e., over the 90th percentile. Therefore, one may conceptualize this phenomenon as a "biologic normalization" process, and a slight deceleration of height growth may not be a harmful consequence of dietary modification.

VI.   Summary

Obesity management is traditionally viewed as a difficult and often unrewarding clinical problem. There may be hesitancy to restrict dietary intake in rapidly growing children because of their relatively high nutritional requirements. Thus, dietary restriction could be viewed as a potentially harmful therapy. Approaches to the clinical evaluation of childhood obesity have been highly variable from physician to physician. Our experience at Duke suggests that caloric restriction can be used to effect weight loss without any untoward effects on growth and development. The systematic schema for clinical evaluation which we have developed at Duke may be helpful to other pediatricians in the comprehensive management of obese children seen in primary care settings.

References

Aristimuno, G. G., Foster, T. A., Voors, A., Srinivasan, S. R. & Berenson, G. S. (1984). Influence of persistent obesity in children on cardiovascular risk factors: The Bogalusa Heart Study. *Circulation* 69:895–904.

Berenson, G. S., Frank, G. C., Hunter, S. M., Srinavasan, S. R., Voors, A. W. & Webber, L. S. (1982). Cardiovascular risk factors in children: should they concern the pediatrician? *Am. J. Dis. Childh.* 136:855–862.

Bjorntorp, P. (1985). Obesity and the risk of cardiovascular disease. *Ann. Clin. Research* 17:3–9.

Bray, G. A. (1985). Complications of obesity. *Ann. Intern. Med.* 103:1052–1062.

Dietz, W. H. (1983). Childhood obesity: Susceptibility, cause, and management. *J. Pediatr.* 103:676–686.

Dietz, W. H. & Hartung, R. (1985). Changes in height velocity of obese preadolescents during weight reduction. *Am. J. Dis. Childh.* 139:705–707.

Forbes, G. B. (1964). Lean body mass and fat in obese children. *Pediatrics* 34:308–314.

Foster, W. R. & Burton, B. T. (Eds.) (1985). Health implications of obesity: National Institutes of Health Consensus Development Conference. *Ann Intern Med.* 103:1068–1077.

Friedman, D. S., Burke, G. L., Harsha, D. W., Srinivasan, S. R., Cresanta, J. L., Webber, L. S. & Berenson, G. S. (1985). Relationship of changes in obesity to serum lipid and lipoprotein changes in childhood and adolescence. *JAMA* 254:515–520.

Fripp, R. R., Hodgson, J. L., Kwiterovich, P. O., Werner, J. C., Schuler, G. & Whitman, V. (1985). Aerobic capacity, obesity, and atherosclerotic risk factors in male adolescents. *Pediatrics* 75:813−818.

Frisancho, A. R. (1981). New norms of upper limb fat and muscle areas for assessment of nutritional status. *Am. J. Clin. Nutr.* 34:2540−2545.

Garfinkel, L. (1985). Overweight and cancer. *Ann. Intern. Med.* 103:1034−1036.

Garn, S. M. (1985). Two-decade follow-up of fatness in early childhood. *Am. J. Dis. Childh.* 139:181−185.

Garn, S. M. & Haskell, J. A. (1960). Fat thickness and developmental status in childhood and adolescence. *Am. J. Dis. Childh.* 99:746−751.

Garrison, R. J. & Castelli, W. P. (1985). Weight and thirty-year mortality of men in the Framingham Study. *Ann. Intern. Med.* 103:1006−1009.

Johnston, F. E. (1985). Health implications of childhood obesity. *Ann. Intern. Med.* 103:1068−1072.

Kelsey, J. L., Acheson, R. M. & Kegg, K. J. (1972). The body build of patients with slipped capital femoral epiphysis. *Am. J. Dis. Childh.* 124:276−281.

Knittle, J. L., Timmers, K. & Ginsberg-Fellner, F. (1979). The growth of adipose tissue in children and adolescents. *J. Clin. Invest.* 63:239−246.

Lauer, R. M., Clarke, W. R. & Beaglehole, R. (1984). Level, trend, and variability of blood pressure during childhood: The Muscatine Study. *Circulation* 69:242−249.

Litt, I. F., Cuskey, W. R. & Rosenberg, A. (1982). Role of self-esteem and autonomy in determining medication compliance among adolescents with juvenile rheumatoid arthritis. *Pediatrics* 69:15−17.

Lucas, C. P., Estigarriba, J. A., Darga, L. L. & Reaven, G. M. (1985). Insulin and blood pressure in obesity. *Hypertension* 7:702−706.

Lukaski, H. C., Johnson, P. E., Bolonchuk, W. W. & Lykken, G. I. (1985). Assessment of fat-free mass using bioelectrical impedance measurements of the human body. *Am. J. Clin. Nutr.* 41:810−817.

Messerli, F. H. (1982). Cardiovascular effects of obesity and hypertension. *Lancet I*:1165−1168.

Piers, E. (1969). Manual for the Piers-Harris Children's Self Concept Scale (The way I feel about myself), Nashville: Counselor Recordings and Tests.

Piers, E. (1977). The Piers-Harris Children's Self Concept Scale. Research Monograph #1, Nashville: Counselor Recordings and Tests.

Riley, D. J., Santiago, T. V. & Edelman, N. H. (1976). Complications of obesity-hypoventilation syndrome in childhood. *Am. J. Dis. Childh.* 130:671−674.

Wadden, T. A., Foster, G. D., Brownell, K. D. & Finley, E. (1984). Self-concept in obese and normal-weight children. *J. Consult. Clin. Psychol.* 52:1104−1105.

Wadden, T. A. & Stunkard, A. J. (1985). Social and psychological consequences of obesity. *Ann. Intern. Med.* 103:1062−1067.

Van Itallie, T. B. (1985). Health implications of overweight and obesity in the United States. *Ann. Intern. Med.* 103:983−988.

Wolf, T. M., Sklov, M. C., Hunter, S. M., Webber, L. S. & Berenson, G. S. (1982). Factor analytic study of the Piers-Harris Children's Self Concept Scale. *J. Person. Assess.* 46:511−513.

Zack, P. M., Harlan, W. R., Leaverton, P. E. & Cornoni-Huntley, J. (1979). A longitudinal study of body fatness in childhood and adolescence. *J. Pediatr.* 95:126−130.

11

Metabolic Aspects of Dieting

WILLIAM H. DIETZ,
New England Medical Center Hospitals
Boston, Massachusetts

The prevalence of obesity among children and adolescents in the United States is increasing rapidly. Using the 85th percentile triceps skinfold, based on data collected from 6–11-year-old children during the National Health Examination Survey (NHES) Cycle II (1963–65), and from 12–17-year-old adolescents collected during NHES Cycle III (1965–68) we (Gortmaker et al, 1987) examined changes in the prevalence of obesity among children and adolescents studied in the first Health and Nutrition Examination Survey (HANES I, 1971–74) and HANES II (1976–80). Over a 15-year period, the prevalence of obesity increased by 54% among 6–11-year-old children, and by 39% among 12–17-year-old adolescents. For the obese child or adolescent, weight reduction is essential.

The three major areas of concern regarding weight reduction for children and adolescents are the optimal formulation for the preservation of lean body mass during weight reduction; the optimal approach to maximizing fat losses during weight reduction; and the principal factors that promote adherence. In each of these areas, data are limited. Nonetheless, we will consider here that which is known, and outline the areas for further research that follow logically from current knowledge.

I. Diet Therapy

Five important problems have generally been neglected in the design of studies that have examined the effects of hypocaloric dietary therapy on obese patients. These are: 1) the changes in body composition that accompany obesity; 2) failure to control the wide intersubject variability that is either intrinsic to subjects or occurs in response to dietary therapy; 3) inferences drawn from short term studies that may be of limited value to predict long term changes in body composition; 4) inferences regarding the interrelationship of glucose and protein metabolism that are drawn from hormone and substrate levels rather than direct measures of gluconeogenesis and protein catabolism; 5) the role of activity in the preservation of lean body mass. Each of these will be considered in turn below.

A.   Alterations in Body Composition

Our own data, as well as others (Forbes, 1964; Cheek et al., 1970) have shown that up to 50% of excess weight in obese adolescents may be fat free mass (FFM). Such increments will expectedly increase protein requirements, so that an adequate intake for an ideal body weight (IBW) for height determined from growth charts may only be of borderline adequacy for an obese patient with a marked increase in FFM. Furthermore, because differences in protein intake alone may affect nitrogen balance, variations in FFM may have been an unrecognized source of error in studies involving small numbers of subjects.

For the present, these observations emphasize that studies of hypocaloric dietary therapy should base protein intakes on lean body mass, measured by one of the techniques used to determine body composition. These data also emphasize the need for reliable anthropometric indicators of lean body mass, suitable for use in clinical settings where measures of body composition are expensive, tedious, or time consuming to perform.

B.   Intersubject Variability

As already stated, lean body mass may vary widely among obese adolescents. Such differences may alter metabolic rate, as well as the reduction in metabolic rate that occurs in response to hypocaloric dietary intakes. In addition, variations in glucose tolerance may alter substrate availability or utilization under normal or hypocaloric conditions.

Under conditions in which wide variation exists between subjects, or occurs in response to an experimental maneuver, or under conditions in which the stage of a disease differs substantially, it is widely accepted that the most valid experimental design is a crossover in which each subject acts as his own control (Snedecor and Cochran, 1980; Cochran and Cox, 1957). Nonetheless, only three previous studies of dietary therapy, two in adults (Yang and Van Itallie, 1976; DeHaven et al., 1980) and our own in adolescents (Dietz and Schoeller, 1982) have used a crossover design.

C.   Study Design

Most studies of hypocaloric dietary therapy have been of short duration, have relied on measures of nitrogen balance rather than more dynamic measures of protein metabolism to evaluate the effects of the diet on lean body mass, and have rarely examined changes in body composition.

The majority of reports of dietary therapy have been conducted over four−six-week periods. The changes in lean body mass that occur during these periods are not markedly greater than the variance of the measures of body composition. In addition, because glycogen contains water, and water content affects every determination of lean body mass except nitrogen measured by neutron activation, diets that alter glycogen content will also affect measures of lean body mass.

Several long-term studies of hypocaloric diets in obese adolescents have recently been made. Over a five-month period, losses of lean body mass accounted for 25% of the weight lost on a diet containing 1.5 gm protein/kg of ideal weight (apparently based on growth charts) .d (Brown et al., 1983). Growth rates in these subjects appeared sub-normal, although the study was short-term, and the season was not specified.

In a second study, conducted over a three-month period in adolescents receiving 2.5 gm protein/kg ideal body weight/day (Archibald et al., 1983) total body nitrogen losses measured by neutron activation were 4.8% (not significant). Total body potassium decreased, as could be predicted from the low carbohydrate content of the diet, which probably produced glycogen losses.

In a third study, we examined the effect of a balanced caloric deficit diet on growth velocity in pre-adolescents studied for a mean of 9.7 months (Dietz and Hartung, 1985). Although growth is not a direct measure of lean body mass, it may be a useful surrogate measure. In this population, growth velocity prior to the introduction of the diet was two standard deviations above the norm in 11 of 19 children. During weight reduction, the decrease in growth velocity was directly related to the change in weight, although growth velocity decreased more than two S. D. below the norm in three patients. The interpretation of these data remains unclear, because the effect of the weight loss was to normalize growth velocity. Nonetheless, these observations stress the importance of monitoring growth velocity during long-term weight reduction, and the need for biochemical measures of protein nutriture in children in whom growth velocity is reduced.

D.   Interrelationships of Protein and Glucose Metabolism

1. *Nitrogen balance in adolescents.*   Despite the high prevalence and morbidity of obesity in adolescents, few published studies have critically compared the effects of hypocaloric diets on nitrogen balance (N-bal). Aside from our previous study (Dietz and Schoeller, 1982; Dietz and Wolfe, 1985) none have utilized a crossover design, and all have relied on limited numbers of subjects (Brown et al., 1983; Archibald, Harrison and Pencharz, 1983; Heald and Hunt, 1965; Merritt et al., 1980; Pencharz et al., 1980). The earliest of these descriptive studies evaluated nitrogen balance in 12 adolescents consuming 1.4−3.0 gm meat protein/kg IBW/day (Merritt et al., 1980). In this study, as well as in a second comparison (Pencharz et al., 1980) of 1.5 gm animal protein plus 20 gm of carbohydrate, several subjects had substantial nitrogen losses that persisted for the duration of the study, and were accompanied by significant decreases in C_3, transferrin, and abumin. One subject developed lymphopenia.

More recently, during a hypocaloric diet providing 1.5 gm protein/kg IBW.d and 500−700 kcal with 28% carbohydrate, losses of lean body mass accounted for 36% of the weight lost in the first five weeks of the diet, and 10% of the weight lost over the next four months (Brown et al., 1983). A final study, using 2.5 gm protein/kg IBW.d, and a mean of 880 kcal with carbohydrate supplying 7% of calories (Archibald et al., 1983), total body nitrogen loss was 5% over a three-month period. Our study of 14 adolescents (Dietz and Schoeller, 1982; Dietz and Wolfe, 1985), compared N-bal for two non-consecutive 21-day periods, preceded by a three-week period of weight maintenance. Protein intake was controlled for FFM. Nitrogen balance was significantly greater when subjects were fed protein plus glucose than when they were fed protein plus fat. Weight losses on the two diets did not differ significantly even when corrected for the losses of fat-free mass calculated from N-balance.

This brief review allows several observations. First, although the data suggest that high protein intakes spare lean body mass, total calories and calories derived from carbohydrates have varied so widely that no firm conclusions can be drawn. Aside from our previous study (Dietz and Schoeller, 1982; Dietz and Wolfe, 1985), all published studies have been descriptive rather than comparative. Finally, in contrast to adults, where N-losses are followed by a plateau or N repletion, adolescents in each of the studies outlined above had persistent N-losses throughout the study period. These observations, in combination with our clinical findings of reduced height velocities in response to balanced calorie deficit diets

(Dietz and Hartung, 1985), emphasize the need for further comparative studies of hypocaloric dietary studies in obese adolescents.

E.   Nitrogen Balance in Adults

In 1974, Flatt and Blackburn (1974) proposed that the low levels of insulin associated with hypocaloric diets free of carbohydrates would increase lipolysis and ketogenesis. The consequent availability of free fatty acids and ketones would diminish glucose utilization, and thereby spare amino acids as precursors for gluconeogenesis.

Studies to test this hypothesis in adults may be summarized as follows (Dietz and Wolfe, 1985): Nitrogen equilibrium or a positive nitrogen balance has been achieved with dietary protein alone (Bistrian et al, 1976; Bistrian et al, 1977; Bistrian, Blackburn and Stanbury, 1977); increased intakes of protein alone will improve nitrogen balance without any effect on insulin, free fatty acids, or ketone bodies (Kekwick and Pawan, 1957; Marliss, Murray, and Nakhooda, 1978); nitrogen balance in patients consuming protein plus glucose does not differ significantly from that observed during feeding of isonitrogenous diets made isocaloric by the addition of fat, but comparisons of insulin, free fatty acids, or ketone bodies were not made (Yang and Van Itallie, 1976); when glucose was added to protein, nitrogen balance improved (Howard et al., 1978) or the quantity of amino acids required for nitrogen balance decreased (Baird, Parsons, and Howard, 1974), despite increases in insulin, or decreases in free fatty acids and ketones (Howard et al, 1978); protein alone compared in a crossover fashion with an isocaloric diet containing protein plus carbohydrate, did not improve nitrogen balance, despite marked increases in ketones and significant decreases in insulin (DeHaven et al., 1980).

All of these studies suffered from the limitations in study design discussed above. None based protein intake on IBW determined by a measurement of body composition. Only two of these studies compared isonitrogenous hypocaloric mixed (Yang and Van Itallie, 1976) or ketogenic diets (DeHaven et al., 1980) in a crossover fashion; no differences in nitrogen balance were observed. Finally the relationship of protein catabolism to glucose production during hypocaloric dietary therapy was inferred rather than measured directly.

F.   Problems with Nitrogen Balance

Nitrogen balance has been the most commonly used short-term measure to assess the adequacy of dietary protein intake. As discussed in detail elsewhere (Hegsted, 1976), this method suffers several difficulties. First, unmeasured losses in protein intake, and unmeasured losses because of incomplete collections are additive. Both will make nitrogen balance appear more positive than is actually the case. Second, perhaps because of these problems, nitrogen balance improves as protein intake increases. This relationship often produces highly questionable results. For example, in a preliminary four-week study comparing nitrogen balance in adolescents consuming (1.5 gm protein + 1.0 gm glucose)/kg IBW.d or 2.5 gm protein /kg IBW.d, we observed that nitrogen balance was considerably more positive on the diet containing protein alone. However, the results also indicated that adolescents gained over 1.0 kg in lean body mass as they were losing weight. This is a highly unlikely result. Finally, nitrogen balance represents net protein catabolism or anabolism. It is not possible to determine from a negative nitrogen balance whether the results represent a decrease in whole body protein synthesis, an increase in whole body protein catabolism, or alterations in both.

These difficulties can be partially resolved by using primed constant infusions of amino acids labeled with stable isotope tracers such as ^{13}C or ^{15}N to measure rates of whole body protein synthesis and catabolism. However, such measures are usually limited to either the fed or fasted state, and are applied for periods of hours rather than days. In addition the rates of protein turnover calculated from these methods depend on the assumption that the size and utilization of the intracellular pools are constant under different dietary conditions. This assumption has not been rigorously tested.

G. Interrelationships of Glucose and Protein Metabolism

Our previous studies have sought to rectify several of the problems outlined above. In a crossover comparison of protein plus glucose with protein plus fat (Dietz and Wolfe, 1985), we measured the interrelationship of new glucose production, determined by U-^{13}C-glucose, and protein catabolism, determined by α-^{15}N-lysine and N-bal.

The interrelationship of protein and glucose metabolism appeared highly dependent on the presence or absence of dietary carbohydrates. Without dietary carbohydrate, rates of glucose production varied directly with nitrogen losses; as nitrogen losses increased, glucose production decreased. These results suggest that N-balance in the absence of dietary carbohydrates is a consequence of net protein catabolism that is not directly mediated by or related to the need for gluconeogenic precursors. In the presence of dietary carbohydrate, nitrogen losses were independent of glucose production, but varied directly with insulin levels. Carbohydrates appeared to reduce net protein catabolism, perhaps by the insulin mediated reduction of amino acid release from skeletal muscle (Pozefsky, 1969) or by the direct stimulation of protein synthesis (Sims et al, 1979). These data also suggest that dietary carbohydrate may maintain body glycogen stores, and thereby buffer glucose production and protein catabolism.

One important source of error is the choice of isotopic label. Use of the ^{13}C glucose label measures total glucose release, but recycling is included in this estimate. Use of the ^2H-glucose label will not include recycled glucose, and estimates of glucose production using ^2H label are approximately 10–30% lower, depending on the metabolic state.

As the only means of establishing a caloric deficit, exercise is less effective than a hypocaloric diet. For example, maximal activity will utilize 300–400 kcal/hour. The likelihood is low that an obese child or adolescent will be able to exercise at this level and will be able to sustain this level of activity for the period of time necessary to lose the excess weight.

However, exercise has a recognized trophic effect on muscle, the largest component of lean body mass. Nonetheless, the effect of exercise, either alone or in combination with hypocaloric dietary therapy, on nitrogen balance, protein metabolism or changes in body composition during weight loss has not been carefully examined in children or adolescents.

II. Fat Losses

Virtually all research into hypocaloric dietary therapy, in both adolescents and adults, has focused on the effects of a hypocaloric diet on nitrogen balance or body composition. Which diet is optimal for maximizing losses of fat remains unclear. Therefore, the effects of diet composition on the adaptation of metabolic rate to a hypocaloric dietary intake appears to be a fruitful area for further research. The comparison of protein alone with protein plus carbohydrate would appear the most interesting investigation, because of the known effects of carbohydrate ingestion on the activity of the sympathetic nervous system.

However, the appropriate method for the demonstration of the likely small differences between these diets remains unclear. Open circuit indirect calorimetry is the most widely available technique to study basal metabolic rate (BMR) and the thermic effects of food (TEF), whereas the doubly labeled water ($^2H_2{}^{18}O$) method is the method of choice for measuring energy expenditure over longer time periods. Both BMR and TEF must be measured, because it is not clear whether the differences anticipated would occur in the fed or fasted state. Likewise, an integrated measure of energy expenditure over time, might help to determine whether the diets influenced activity. The most general approach would be to examine the proportion of total daily energy expenditure not attributable to BMR. This latter expression affords an integrated indirect assessment of TEF and activity. However, measurement of total daily energy expenditure is expensive and requires highly sophisticated analytic equipment that is not widely available or utilized for this purpose. Furthermore, because substantial interindividual variation is likely in the metabolic adaptation to weight reduction, crossover designs are essential. Such a design further increases the difficulty of such studies.

III. Adherence

Although it is popularly believed that the choice of the diet is the key to the likelihood of successful weight reduction, few data support this assumption. We have now studied over 40 subjects who followed either a ketotic or carbohydrate-containing diet after discharge from the MIT Clinical Research Center. On both diets, the success of long-term weight maintenance at a reduced weight was low and did not differ. These observations suggest that to some extent, considerations regarding the prevention of losses of FFM and fat are irrelevant to the long term success of weight reduction. Factors that promote adherence therefore require more intensive investigation.

Our experience has been that family factors are the most significant variables that affect the success of hypocaloric diets in children and adolescents. Data supporting this experience are derived from three sources. First, the association of family variables with obesity in children and adolescents has been widely recognized. These associations include parental obesity, socioeconomic class, education, marital status, family size, birth order and television viewing (Dietz and Gortmaker, 1984; Dietz and Gortmaker, 1985). Second, we have shown (Dietz, 1983) that both marital status and parental obesity are independently associated with rates of weight reduction. In addition, a program involving both parents and child together was more successful than a program that treated parents and children separately (Brownell, Kelman, and Stunkard, 1983). Finally, in collaboration with Jill Harkaway, we have demonstrated highly reproducible interactive sequences within families. For example, in families of obese adolescents in which one parent is also obese, covert conflict between the parents about the obese parent's weight often exists. This conflict often presents a conflict about the adolescent's weight and disagreement about the optimal means for weight reduction. Under such circumstances, the adolescent's obesity maintains family homeostasis. Weight loss risks an overt conflict between the parents.

Our understanding of these relationships is still rudimentary. Nonetheless, the association of family variables with both the onset and course of obesity suggests that the causes of obesity and its persistence may be similar. The development of quantitative means to assess these interactions is crucial to the next step in the description of such families, and testing whether the alteration of these patterns effects successful weight reduction.

References

Archibald, E. H., Harrison, J. W. E., Pencharz, P.B. (1983). Effect of a weight-reducing high-protein diet on the body composition of obese adolescents. *Am. J. Dis. Childh.,* *137*:658−662.

Baird, I. M., Parsons, R. L., Howard, A. N. (1974). Clinical and metabolic studies of chemically defined diets in the management of obesity. *Metabolism, 23*:645.

Bistrian, B. R., Winterer, J., Blackburn, G. L., Young, V. R. & Sherman, M. (1977). Effect of a protein-sparing diet and brief fast on nitrogen metabolism in mildly obese subjects. *J. Lab. Clin. Med., 89*:1030.

Bistrian, B. R., Blackburn, G. L., Stanbury, J. B. (1977). Metabolic aspects of a protein-sparing modified fast in the dietary management of Prader-Willi obesity. *N. Engl. J. Med., 296*:744−749.

Bistrian, B. R., Blackburn G. L., Flatt, J.-P., Sizer, J., Scrimshaw, N. S., Sherman, M. (1976). Nitrogen metabolism and insulin requirements in obese diabetic adults on a protein-sparing modified fast. *Diabetes, 25*:494−504.

Brown, M. R., Klish, W. J., Hollander, J., Campbell M. A., Forbes, G. B. (1983). A high protein, low calorie liquid diet in the treatment of very obese adolescents: Long-term effect on lean body mass. *Am. J. Clin. Nutr., 38*:20−31.

Brownell, K. D., Kelman, J. H., Stunkard, A. M. (1983). Treatment of obese children with and without their mothers: Changes in weight and blood pressure. *Pediatrics, 71*:515−523.

Cheek, D. B., Schultz, R. B., Parra, A., Reba, R. C. (1970). Overgrowth of lean and adipose tissue in adolescent obesity. *Pediatr. Res., 4*:268−279.

Cochran, W. B., Cox, G. M. (1957). *Experimental Designs* (2nd ed.). New York: John Wiley and Sons, Inc.,

DeHaven, J., Sherwin, R., Hendler, R. & Felig, P. (1980). Nitrogen and sodium balance and sympathetic-nervous system activity in obese subjects treated with a low-calorie protein or mixed diet. *N. Engl. J. Med., 302*:477−482.

Dietz, W. H., Schoeller, D. A. (1982). Optimal dietary therapy for obese adolescents: Comparison of protein plus glucose and protein plus fat. *J. Pediatr., 100*:638−644.

Dietz, W. H., Jr. (1983). Family characteristics affect rates of weight loss in obese children. *Nutr. Res., 3*:43−50.

Dietz, W. H., Gortmaker, S. L. (1984). Epidemiologic variables associated with childhood obesity. *J. Am. Coll. Nutr. 3*:267.

Dietz, W. H., Hartung, R. (1985). Changes in height velocity of obese preadolescents during weight reduction. *Am. J. Dis. Childh., 139*:705−707.

Dietz, W. H., Wolfe, R. R. (1985). Interrelationships of glucose and protein metabolism during hypocaloric dietary therapy in obese adolescents. *Am. J. Clin. Nutr., 42*:380−390.

Dietz, W. H., Gortmaker S. L. (1985). Do we fatten our children at the TV set? Obesity and television viewing in children. *Pediatrics, 75*:807−812.

Gortmaker, S. L., Dietz, W. H., Sobol, A. M., Wehler, C. A. (1987). Trends in the prevalence of childhood and adolescent obesity in the United States. *Am. J. Dis. Childh., 141*:535–540.

Flatt, J. P., Blackburn, G. L. (1974). The metabolic fuel regulatory system: Implications for protein sparing therapies during caloric deprivation and disease. *Am. J. Clin. Nutr., 27*:175–187.

Forbes, G. B. (1964). Lean body mass and fat in obese children. *Pediatrics, 34*:308–314.

Heald, F. P., Hunt, S. M. (1965). Caloric dependency in obese adolescents is affected by degree of maturation. *J. Pediatr., 66*:1035–41.

Hegsted, M. (1976). Balance Studies. *J. Nutr. 106*:307–314.

Howard, L., Dobs, A., Chados, R., Chu, R. & Toludice, T. (1978). A comparison of administering protein alone and protein plus glucose on nitrogen balance. *Am. J. Clin. Nutr., 31*:226.

Kekwick, A., Pawan, G. L. S. (1957). Metabolic study in human obesity with isocaloric diets high in fat, protein, or carbohydrate. *Metabolism, 6*:447–460.

Marliss, E. B., Murray, F. T. & Nakhooda, A. G. (1978). The metabolic response to hypocaloric protein diets in obese man. *J. Clin. Invest., 62*:468–479.

Merritt, R. J., Bistrian, B. R., Blackburn, G. L., Suskind, R. M. (1980). Consequences of modified fasting in obese pediatric and adolescent patients. I. Protein-sparing modified fast. *J. Pediatr., 96*:13–19.

Pencharz, P. B., Motil, K. J., Parsons, H. G. & Duffy, B. J. (1980). The effect of an energy-restricted diet on the protein metabolism of obese adolescent patients: nitrogen balance and whole-body nitrogen turnover. *Clin. Sci. 59*:13–18.

Pozefsky, T., Felig, P., Tobin, J. D., Soeldner, S., Cahill, G. F. (1969). Amino acid balance across tissues of the forearm in post-absorptive man. Effects of insulin at two dose levels. *J. Clin. Invest., 48*:2273–2282.

Sims, A. J. W., Wolfe, M. B., Young, V. R., Clarke, D., Moore, F. D. (1979). Glucose promotes whole body synthesis from infused amino acids in fasting man. *Lancet, 1*:68–71.

Snedecor, G. W. & Cochrane, W. G., (1980). *Statistical Methods* (7th ed.) Ames Iowa, Iowa State University Press.

Yang, M.-U., Van Itallie, T. B. (1976). Composition of weight lost during short-term weight reduction. *J. Clin. Invest., 58*:722–730.

12

Parental and Family Influences in the Etiology and Treatment of Childhood Obesity

ALLEN C. ISRAEL
Department of Psychology
University at Albany, State University of New York
Albany, New York

I. Introduction

The problem of obesity was one focus of early research on behavioral treatments. This choice, and it was largely adult research, was made for a number of reasons. Among these were some that, from our current perspective, seem naive. It was expected that the obesity problem presented a therapeutic target that was easily and objectively measured — a rarity in psychological treatment research. Even at its most basic level, this was oversimplified. Furthermore, the logic of the behavioral approach has led us to realize that one faces a difficult task in measuring the environmental variables and real−life behaviors we need to evaluate in our treatment research. Those who undertook obesity research because it was a simple, straightforward problem of easily changed habits were quickly educated by their patients or research participants (cf Foreyt and Kondo, 1984; Israel & Stolmaker, 1980).

It seems clearer to us now that obesity is a complex problem that will require far more professional effort and creativity (cf. Stunkard, 1980; Wooley, Wooley, and Dyrenforth, 1979). It is not an issue of genetics vs. failures of willpower or defensive eating. Rather the problem is clearly one that requires the perspective of a biobehavioral transaction. It is not wise to look for unitary causal explanations or simple treatments that fit all cases. Rather, one is required to be able to be flexible, and research the level at which one deals with the problem; to be able to address the individuality of a particular case while being able to see the commonalities that advance knowledge; and to appreciate the ongoing complex transactions between biological, person, immediate environmental, and social—cultural issues, while being able to focus attention on one particular aspect. This transition from the contextual whole to a particular piece and back again goes on at multiple levels and is not a simple task. As our knowledge of childhood obesity progresses, and as the implications of one piece for the other become clearer, it is to be hoped that this task will become an easier one. Both the practitioner and the researcher will, however, continue to be required to appreciate the "larger" context without the embarrassment of taking a "smaller" focus and to take this smaller focus without arrogance or blindness to the larger whole.

Indeed, the challenge of any one contribution to a volume, such as this one, is similar — keeping a larger picture, but focusing on a particular piece or pieces. This is based on the arguable assumption that advancement of knowledge and practice will be best served by researchers who are able to think in large contextual terms and at the same time be able to focus on a piece of the puzzle.

This contribution arises from a particular focus — the behavioral management of childhood obesity — and in this chapter on the role of parent/family influences. Many of the questions asked and directions offered arise from the kinds of transitions of thinking described above. This process is not always visible. The larger volume is a chance to view the whole. The focus here is on one segment of the puzzle and on one approach to working with it.

II. Parental Involvement in the Treatment Process

The importance of parental involvement in the treatment of obese children is supported by both logic and empirical evidence. An emphasis on the parental role can also be appreciated in the context of work on other childhood problems (e.g., Forehand, and McMahon, 1981; Patterson, 1986) and the role of significant others in management of adult obesity (e.g., Brownell, Heckerman, Westlake, Hayes, and Monti, 1978; Foreyt and Kondo, 1984; Israel and Saccone, 1979). Epidemiological examinations of the problem of childhood obesity are clearly consistent with the centrality of family environment in both the etiology and treatment of the disorder (e.g., Dietz, 1983; Khoury, Morrison, Laskarzewski, and Glueck, 1983). The task of unraveling these influences at an operational level and in a manner that allows reliable and valid measurement is clearly a complex one. There are, however, guidelines for involvement in such an endeavor.

Particularly for the young child, the parent is centrally involved in food preparation and availability. Parents are also likely to be central in establishing knowledge of nutrition as well as attitudes towards and patterns of food consumption (cf. Harper and Sanders, 1975; Klesges et al., 1983; Klesges, Malott, Boschee, and Weber, 1986; Laskarzewski et al., 1980; Rozin, Fallon, and Mandell, 1984). This, of course, is only half of the energy balance equation. The parents' role in the child's activity level and energy expenditure, although often given less attention, demands addressing as well (e.g., Klesges et al., 1984; Klesges et al., 1986). Finally, any attempt to work with the obese child will in some way involve the parent in the task of managing the child's behavior and achieving a developmentally appropriate level of parental control and child self-control. The parent is likely to be involved in various roles already: Controller of environment, model of behavior (in its broadest sense), and regulator of behavior (e.g., Birch, Marlin, and Rotter, 1984; Harper and Sanders, 1975; Klesges et al., 1983; Klesges et al., 1984; Klesges et al., 1986).

The logic and contextual empirical support of parent involvement needs to be applied to treatment programs for obese children. This leads one to the task of articulating family environmental influences. One must then create mechanisms for addressing these influences in the design of prevention and treatment programs. At minimum this would seem to involve assuring parental involvement. How such involvement is implemented and defined is clearly an issue worthy of research attention.

Perhaps the most direct definition of this involvement is parental attendance/participation in treatment. Indeed, to date, most behavioral programs have included parents in treatment. Kingsley and Shapiro (1977) experimentally defined parental involvement as attendance at sessions. Their study compared the weight loss of children who attended sessions with their mother, children who attended alone and whose mothers received handouts, and children whose mothers attended sessions without them. While the mother-child group tended to do best during follow-up, there were no significant differences between groups during either treatment or follow-up. More recently, Brownell and his colleagues have demonstrated that employing separate groups for parents and adolescents produced greater weight loss and maintenance than did groups which included the mother and adolescent together or a condition in which the adolescents were seen but parents were not involved (Brownell, Kelman, and Stunkard, 1983). These findings also alert us to possible developmental aspects of parental involvement (Harris and Ferrari, 1983; Israel, Stolmaker, Sharp, Silverman, and Simon, 1984).

One can also attempt to distinguish aspects of the attendance/participation dimension. For example, Kirschenbaum, Harris, and Tomarken (1984) compared two different parental attendance conditions, one in which the child and parent attended together versus one in which the child attended alone but the parent participated through printed handouts covering the same material, homework, and home discussions with the child. There were no differences in the children's success at weight loss between the two conditions. However, the parental "participation/non-attendance" condition did result in greater rates of attrition.

In contrast, one can vary only the participation portion of this construct. For example, Epstein and his colleagues (Epstein, Wing, Koeske, Andrasik, and Ossip, 1981) had all parents attend, but variation in contingencies addressed the question of parental participation. Interventions were applied to both parent's and child's weight loss, child's weight loss alone, or to a nonspecific target. Again, while no overall group differences emerged, a significant correlation between parent's and child's weight loss during treatment was reported. In addition, there was an indication that successful children in the parent/child condition exhibited better maintenance.

In our own work we have started from the level of parental involvement being defined by regular attendance and participation (the targeting of parent as well as child behavior change). The results of the above research do not always clearly support the additional targeting of the parent. However, the available evidence suggests this direction. Further, the logic of such a strategy leads us to attribute the lack of significant differences, where they occur, to the particular definitions of parental intervention employed. This then suggests the exploration of alternative strategies for targeting parental change.

Two aspects of the parental involvement concept seemed quite salient to us. The first was, how were parents to be involved? That is, how would their role be implemented in the treatment process — how would *their* behavior be targeted for change. Many programs involve parents by expecting them to engage in their own weight loss effort. This is clearly a logical implementation and a potentially successful one (e.g., Epstein et al., 1981). There are, however, two possible limitations to this approach. The more obvious is, by definition, that this limits involvement to families with an overweight participating parent. The other relates to the advisability, in all cases, of employing parental weight loss as the mechanism of change. A family behavior change focus suggests sensitivity to certain questions. For example, what is the potential impact of parental failure or relapse in instances where the family's change has been defined as parallel weight loss? Interpersonal issues such as parent-child competition/comparison and the need for the child to feel she is receiving special attention may also arise from broader clinical considerations. Indeed, these issues may be raised by the families themselves.

These considerations suggest that while parental change is a necessary focus, it may be necessary to consider strategies other than parental weight loss. This, of course, does not indicate abandoning the parental weight loss mechanism. Rather, the availability of an alternative focus is suggested. A "natural" alternative to parental weight loss is to define explicitly parental change in the helper role. This strategy is natural in that asking the parent to serve as a change agent (helper) is inherent in most existing behavioral interventions. The issue is then one of emphasis and the explicitness of this focus.

We undertook a comparison of these two mechanisms for ensuring parental involvement and targeting behavior change (Israel et al., 1984). The helper and weight loss roles for parents were compared in a multi-faceted behavioral treatment program for overweight children between 8 and 12 years of age. The weight loss role asked parents to engage in their own weight loss effort. Explicit parental weight reduction assignments and behavior change targets paralleled those of the child and were clearly explicated as the focus of the parents own behavior change efforts. In contrast, while the program was structured to have all participating parents assist the child in her/his weight loss efforts, parents in the helper role had this task more clearly explicated. That is, their assignments, monitoring, and behavior change targets focused on these helping behaviors. Thus, both sets of parents were, necessarily, involved in their child's weight loss efforts. For one group, however, greater emphasis was given to this role and this was *the* focus of their behavior change. We elected to allow families to select which of the two roles they preferred. The selection was done in consultation with program personnel. This procedure was chosen for several reasons. It provides the greatest external validity to non-research clinical application. Furthermore, it seemed most consistent with the conceptual rationale for exploring the two roles. Also, random assignment to a role might not be viewed as a neutral process in research instances such as the present one, and thus the intended control would not be achieved. Finally, weight loss by a normal weight or underweight parent would be inappropriate.

At the end of the treatment period children in the helper and weight loss conditions had achieved comparable weight reductions. In contrast, waiting list controls had experienced a weight gain. Similarly, at one-year follow-up the two conditions were not significantly different either in terms of change in percent overweight, number of successful maintainers, or children reaching non-obese status. The results of this program, like most others, did point to the need for improved treatment and maintenance strategies. In the present context, however, it would appear that both parental involvement roles are equally efficacious. One potential criticism of the above findings was the brief period that parents were supervised in their respective roles. In a subsequent investigation, the helper and weight loss roles were compared over an extended treatment period of approximately six months (Israel, Solotar, and Zimand, 1986). Again, the two parental involvement conditions produced equivalent changes in child percent overweight during both the treatment and follow-up periods. These results provide an extended replication of earlier findings.

One qualification of the above conclusion may, however, also be suggested by the earlier findings. A pattern emerged whereby, during treatment, the helper role may have been more successful for older children (10−12 years of age) while, during the follow-up period, no differences between roles were suggested for this age group. Younger children (8−10 years of age), however, may have benefited more with the weight-loss role during both periods. Small expected values prohibited statistical comparisons of these data, and the small sample sizes suggest considerable caution in drawing conclusions. The findings are consistent, however, with being sensitive to developmental issues in implementing parental involvement, or indeed any intervention.

Before moving on from the issue of the weight loss/helper aspects of parental involvement, one other finding is worth noting. A number of investigators have reported greater correlations between child and parent weight change during periods of reduced contact or follow-up than is the case during treatment itself (e.g., Epstein, Wing, Koeske, and Valoski, 1985; Israel et al., 1985, 1986). Particularly intriguing is the finding by Kirschenbaum et al. (1984) that when parents attended sessions, this pattern occurred, as in the above research, as a positive correlation. However, when the parents did not attend, the relationship between parent and child success was an inverse one. Clearly in evaluating parental involvement, the complexity of long-term considerations must be given serious attention. At present, however, a clear understanding of how the relationship operates between parental and child change during this period is unavailable and thus a priority. That the relationship is not a simple one is suggested not only by the above results, but also by the difficulty, to date, in achieving consistent long-term success.

III. Parenting Skills

A somewhat different aspect of the parental involvement issue is the ability to apply the parenting skills necessary for implementing child behavior change. One of the early behavioral treatment studies provides a suggestion of the importance of addressing these skills. Aragona, Cassady, and Drabman (1975) compared two conditions for consequating changes. A response cost plus reinforcement condition was compared to response cost alone. However, parents in the first group were also provided with some training in general child management skills. Analysis of the outcome of these interventions employing a weight reduction index (Edwards, 1978) suggested better maintenance in the combined condition. While small sample size and other considerations suggest caution in drawing conclusions, these results and the logic of behavioral interventions are consistent with the view that explicit attention to child management skills is likely to facilitate sustained weight loss by the child.

Israel, Stolmaker, and Andrian (1985) directly addressed this question. Overweight children, 8 to 12 years of age and their parents were assigned to one of two treatment conditions or a waiting list control. Participants in the Weight Reduction Only (WRO) condition received a multifaceted behavioral treatment program which required the parents to be directly involved in their child's weight loss efforts. These parents, in addition to receiving instructions in all areas, were required to define problem behaviors, monitor and consequate behaviors and were instructed and guided in this procedure. Thus, training in child management skills was inherent and addressed to this condition. However, parents in the Parent Training (PT) condition received this "standard" program but also had training in child management skills enhanced and emphasized. Prior to the start of the weight reduction program, parents in the PT condition read a child management text and attended two sessions in which they were instructed in behavioral child management skills. Concepts presented during the parent training sessions were systematically referred to during the ensuing treatment program. Other than the text, the two-session course, and continued review of child management principles, the two groups received identical treatment.

Both treatments were superior to the control condition and resulted in equivalent absolute weight loss and comparable numbers of children meeting prescribed weekly weight loss goals. However, WRO children achieved a greater reduction in percent overweight than did the PT children. During the period between the end of treatment and a one-year follow-up, however, children in the PT condition evidenced a nonsignificant mean decrease in percent overweight, whereas WRO children exhibited a significant mean increase. Thus, while the groups were probably comparable during treatment, there is the suggestion of better maintenance even with a relatively small increment in child management skills training. This conclusion is reinforced by analyses of the parent's child management knowledge (KBPAC — O'Dell, Tarler-Benlolo, and Flynn, 1979). These results indicated that PT parents had achieved greater knowledge of these principles by the end of treatment. There was not, however, a significant correlation between KBPAC scores and change in the child's weight status during treatment. At the one-year follow-up, PT parents maintained their higher KBPAC scores. Also higher scores at this point appeared to be related to greater success in the child's weight loss effort over the entire period from beginning of treatment through follow-up.

These findings suggest that explicit training in child management skills enhances knowledge, that the impact of such training appears to be sustained, and that such knowledge may have long-term implications regarding the child's success. Clearly, these results directly address only the parent's knowledge of these principles. Actual measurement of parenting skills would clearly enhance our understanding. However, the obtained relationship to long-term outcome and the condition differences are consistent with the conclusion that this knowledge is being translated into action by parents.

IV. Family Variables as Predictors of Outcome

Another strategy for articulating family issues is to assess attributes of families of obese children who present for treatment. This is a somewhat different strategy than one which examines the relationship between certain variables and the prevalence of a problem. The strategy described here seeks to examine family variables as they are related to the treatment process. However, this is done in a way that is likely to inform our understanding of the development of the problem as well.

As an attempt to initiate this process, Israel, Silverman, and Solotar (1986) examined a number of attributes of families seeking behavioral treatment for their overweight child. The selection of potential variables was guided by several considerations including current ability to define and measure the attribute clearly, previous clinical or empirical literature suggesting an association, and existing research methodological conventions. In addition to relationships with treatment outcome, the question of who seeks treatment and who prematurely terminates treatment were explored. The impact of well-developed interventions is greatly reduced if a large number of families do not seek treatment or if they drop out of treatment prematurely.

The investigated sample consisted of 91 families with a designated target child. The children ranged in age from 8 years, 0 months to 13 years, 5 months (M = 10 years, 8 months) and were from 21.8 to 99.4%

overweight (M = 49.47) prior to treatment. The family variables of interest in the present study are described below.

Although both parents of intact families were encouraged to attend the treatment sessions, they were given the option of having either the mother or the father attend. Given the importance of the attendance/participation concept, the impact of having either the mother, father, or both parents attend sessions was explored.

Available literature clearly indicates a correlation between parental and child fatness (cf. Dietz, 1983; Epstein and Cluss, 1986). However, variations in weight status among parents of children attending treatment were also salient to us. Based on these observations, the impact on the treatment process of whether the child has zero, one, or two overweight parents was examined.

In addition, earlier work with intact families in our weight-loss programs indicated that there were wide variations in the quality and/or stability of marriages. Therefore, the relationship of marital satisfaction to the children's weight loss effort was explored. The families were also classified according to SES occupational category. The higher status occupation of the two parents was the one included in the classification.

Available data on obese families (e.g., Dietz, 1983; Khoury et al., 1983) and the logic of an environmental-influence model also suggested sibling weight status as another factor that was likely to be of importance. Target children were categorized into one of the following three groups: (1) only child, (2) no overweight sibling(s), or (3) one or more overweight sibling(s). Progress in the program for these three groups was then compared.

In examining the issues of who presents for treatment and the child's initial weight status, a number of interesting findings emerged. These data do not necessarily tell us which family factors "cause" childhood obesity. Also, procedural differences with epidemiological investigations should be kept in mind. These results do, however, give us a better picture of the families who seek services. Attending parent's weight status and SES emerged as significant predictors of child's initial weight status among intact families. For single parent families, parental weight status was again a significant predictor; however, SES was not, but sibling weight status was.

Children of overweight attending parents were found to be heavier than those of non-overweight attending parents. This finding could be taken to suggest nothing more than the well known adage that obesity "runs in families." However, several factors militate against this explanation. The relationship is with degree and not prevalence of childhood obesity. Also, neither the weight status of the non-attending parent nor the number of overweight parents was related to the child's initial degree of overweight. A possible explanation for these findings is that parents of normal weight status may be quicker than overweight parents in seeking professional help when they notice their child gaining excessive weight. That is, they may seek treatment earlier, before the problem becomes severe.

Consistent with this is the finding that while approximately 16% of the children presenting for treatment were only children, and 16% had one or more overweight siblings, 68% had siblings but were the only overweight child. This is in relation to obesity prevalence data suggesting the greater likelihood of overweight siblings and only child families (cf. Dietz, 1983). Perhaps parents are also more likely to notice that their child is overweight and to seek professional help if they have other children who are not overweight and with whom the targeted child may be compared. Conversely, being one of several overweight children may decrease the likelihood of the problem's being seen as one requiring action. It may also be the case that a single overweight child among non-overweight siblings causes greater difficulties for the family system. These stresses and their general impact on the designated child (e.g., Israel and Shapiro, 1985) may lead to seeking assistance. This possible pattern of treatment seeking suggests that families with more than one overweight child need to be reached. That this "sibling influence" is not solely a function of parental weight status (and thus "overweight families") is indicated by the fact that both overweight and non-overweight attending parents had equivalent distributions of only children, only overweight children, and children with one or more overweight siblings.

The finding that children of lower SES families were more overweight prior to treatment than children of middle and higher SES families is consistent with other reports of associations of SES and the prevalence of obesity (e.g., Garn and Clark, 1976). However, it is, again, also possible that this finding with degree of overweight indicates something more. Unlike middle and higher SES families, lower SES families may seek assistance only when their child's weight problem becomes severe. Finally, although approximately 80% of the present sample consisted of intact families, there was no difference in the child's initial percent overweight in these and single-parent homes. Also, among intact families marital satisfaction did not appear to be related to the degree of initial overweight.

If our above speculations, and they are indeed that, are correct, then there are implications regarding particular populations that need to be targeted for preventative or early interventions: specifically, children whose potential attending parent (usually the mother) is overweight, those who have siblings who are also overweight, and those of lower SES status.

Without special efforts, these children may not be entered into treatment until much later in the weight-gain process. Clearly these are not the only variables that may guide prevention efforts, but they do appear to be reasonable ones.

The impact of these family variables on treatment dropout was also assessed. Families of lower SES and of single parent status had the highest dropout rates. The already strained resources of these families probably accounts for their greater rate of attrition, a finding and conceptualization not dissimilar to those noted in other problem areas (e.g., Dumas and Wahler, 1983). In the area of childhood obesity treatment itself, there is some evidence that children whose family environments are characterized as chaotic are more likely to drop out of treatment (Kirschenbaum et al., 1984). Such a conceptualization might suggest making programmatic alterations and providing special assistance to these families, particularly during the initial phase of treatment. Also identification of the variables that make some of these families "invulnerable" to influence causing dropout will inform our understanding of the treatment process in general.

Although the family variables studied do appear to impact on initial weight status and attrition, none of these variables were clearly related to treatment outcome. The present findings apply to within-treatment change and different sets of variables may be related to longer-term change. For example, our findings indicate that parental obesity was unrelated to treatment outcome. Epstein and his colleagues (Epstein, Wing, Koeske, and Valoski, 1986) have also reported no such differences at 3 years following the initiation of treatment. However, their results suggest a more rapid weight gain during follow-up for children of obese parents. Several interesting trends in our findings are, however, worth mentioning — with appropriate caution clearly acknowledged. Children from intact families (but not single-parent families) tended to be more successful if their attending parent was overweight. Also, among extremely successful children, intact families with nonsatisfactory marriages, seemed to be disproportionately represented. An explanation addressing both weight status of the participating parent and marital status might view the parent as the child's advocate. An overweight attending parent may serve as a more cooperative and sympathetic ally especially in an environment where the other parent may be less committed to weight loss or indeed provide environmental influences that run counter to therapeutic goals. This counter influence is reduced or absent in single parent families and may be less relevant to the attending parent from an intact but unsatisfactory marriage. While tentative, this explanation is consistent with our clinical impressions.

There was also a tendency for weight loss to be smaller for children who had siblings but who were the only overweight child. Perhaps the child contrasts the changes that are expected with the relative lack of demands placed upon his or her siblings. Also, there may be real environmental differences. High-calorie snacks made accessible to non-overweight siblings may be a potential obstacle to the obese child. These and related issues are likely to contribute to a more difficult change process for the child who has siblings of normal weight status.

These findings regarding siblings and parental weight status/marital adjustment, are consistent with our clinical impressions that inclusion of the entire family in the treatment plan is a direction worthy of exploration. Beyond the family patterns mentioned above, it is likely that other aspects of family functioning influence outcome. A consistent attitude among family members regarding the child's weight and change is one potential agenda. This attitude, a sense of family cohesiveness, an organization for problem solving, and communication skills seem to be characteristic of many of our successful families. A related issue that impresses us as important is the ability of the parents to adopt a consistent, rather than short-term, parenting style. Both these impressions find some limited empirical support in Kirschenbaum et al.'s (1984) finding of short-term increases in factors such as cohesion, mutual support, and expression of feeling among families undergoing behavioral treatment for childhood obesity. High levels of these qualities were also related to short-term success.

V. Future Directions

While progress is clearly being made, what we need to know remains extensive and varied. Thus, statements of directions for future research must be viewed as suggestions and not limitations. Indeed, diverse and creative thinking seems required. With this caution, it seems possible to identify certain themes within this piece of the puzzle. Clarifying the nature of parental involvement during periods of reduced contact remains a challenge. It is clear that the nature of such involvement will have appreciable impact on long-term success. This in itself is a multifaceted issue. Identifying families that might benefit from different approaches to the parent/child weight loss issue is one aspect of this problem. Parental weight-loss relapse, for example, seems likely given adult findings. Why does this not occur with some parents? If it does, what protects some children from following this pattern? How is it that this relationship may be an inverse one under some circumstances?

We also still need to provide guidelines that are better attuned to general developmental issues. Appropriate parenting skills and a balance between parental and child control (cf., Cohen, Gelfand, Dodd, Jensen, and Turner, 1980) are only some of the areas needing a clearer developmental focus. Identifying and measuring actual situations and parental behaviors that mediate successful long-term change is also a priority. Guidelines are available, but more needs to be known about the specifics of such behavior in successful families.

Finally, the larger family context cannot be ignored. Incorporation of other family members into treatment plans or actual involvement in sessions seems likely to enhance our progress. This is a difficult practical task, but it is also one for which empirical guidelines need to be refined.

That these suggestions stop at these borders should not be taken as an indication that "here is where influence ends." In returning to the larger perspective which opened this contribution, this is a focus on only one piece of the puzzle. As one steps back, there are many other potential themes to explore. One's view of any particular piece the next time one "focuses in" should be altered by having viewed the larger whole.

References

Aragona, J., Cassady, J., & Drabman, R. S. (1975). Treating overweight children through parental training and contingency contracting. *Journal of Applied Behavior Analysis, 8,* 269–278.

Birch, L. L., Marlin, D. W., & Rotter, J. (1984). Eating as the "means" activity in a contingency: Effects on young children's food preference. *Child Development, 55,* 431–439.

Brownell, K. D., Heckerman, C. L., Westlake, R. J., Hayes, S. C., & Monti, P. M. (1978). The effect of couples training partner cooperativeness in the behavioral treatment of obesity. *Behavior Research and Therapy, 16,* 323–333.

Cohen, E., Gelfand, D., Dodd, D., Jensen, J., & Turner, C. (1980). Self-control practices associated with weight loss maintenance in children and adolescents. *Behavior Therapy, 11,* 26–37.

Dietz, W. H., Jr. (1983). Childhood obesity: Susceptibility, causes, and management. *The Journal of Pediatrics, 103,* 676–686.

Dumas, J. E., & Wahler, R. G. (1983). Predictors of treatment outcome in parent training: Mother insularity and socioeconomic disadvantage. *Behavioral Assessment, 5,* 301–313.

Edwards, K. A. (1978). An index for assessing weight changes in children: Weight/height ratios. *Journal of Applied Behavior Analysis, 11,* 421–429.

Epstein, L. H., & Cluss, P. A. (1986). Behavioral genetics of childhood obesity. *Behavior Therapy, 17,* 324–334.

Epstein, L. H., Koeske, R., Wing, R. R., & Valoski, A. (1986). The effect of family variables on child weight change. *Health Psychology, 5(1),* 1–11.

Epstein, L. H., Wing, R. R., Koeske, R., Andrasik, F., & Ossip, D. J. (1981). Child and parent weight loss in family-based behavior modification programs. *Journal of Consulting and Clinical Psychology, 49,* 674–685.

Epstein, L. H., Wing, R. R., Koeske, R., & Valoski, A. (1985). A comparison of life-style exercise, aerobic exercise, and calisthenics on weight loss in obese children. *Behavior Therapy, 16,* 345–356.

Forehand, R., & McMahon, R. J. (1981). *Helping the noncompliant child: A clinician's guide to parent training.* New York: Guilford.

Foreyt, J. P., & Kondo, A. T. (1984). Advances in behavioral treatment of obesity. In M. Hersen, R. M. Eisler, & P. M. Miller (Eds.) *Progress in Behavior Modification,* Volume 16. Orlando: Academic Press, Inc.

Garn, S. M., & Clark, D. C. (1976). Trends in fatness and the origins of obesity. *Pediatrics, 57,* 443–456.

Harper, L. V., & Sanders, K. M. (1975). The effect of adult's eating on young children's acceptance of unfamiliar foods. *Journal of Experimental Child Psychology, 20,* 206–214.

Harris, S. L., & Ferrari, M. (1983). Developmental factors in child behavior therapy. *Behavior Therapy, 14,* 54–72.

Israel, A. C., & Saccone, A. J. (1979). Follow-up of effects of choice of mediator and target of reinforcement on weight loss. *Behavior Therapy, 10,* 260–265.

Israel, A. C., & Shapiro, L. S. (1985). Behavior problems of obese children enrolling in a weight reduction program. *Journal of Pediatric Psychology, 10,* 449–460.

Israel, A. C., Silverman, W. K., & Solotar, L. C. (1986). An investigation of family influences on initial weight status, attrition, and treatment outcome in a childhood obesity program. *Behavior Therapy, 17,* 131–143.

Israel, A. C., Solotar, L. C., & Zimand, E. (1986). *An Extended Examination of Parental Weight Loss and Helper Roles in the Treatment of Childhood Obesity.* Unpublished manuscript.

Israel, A. C., & Stolmaker, L. B. (1980). Behavioral treatment of obesity in children and adolescents. In M. Hersen, R. M. Eisler, & P. M. Miller (Eds.), *Progress in Behavior Modification.* Volume 10. New York: Academic Press.

Israel, A. C., Stolmaker, L., & Andrian, C. A. G. (1985). The effects of training parents in general child management skills on a behavioral weight loss program for children. *Behavior Therapy, 16,* 169–180.

Israel, A. C., Stolmaker, L., Sharp, J. P., Silverman, W. K., & Simon, L. G. (1984). An evaluation of two methods of parental involvement in treating obese children. *Behavior Therapy, 15,* 266–272.

Khoury, P., Morrison, J. A., Laskarzewski, P. M., & Glueck, C. J. (1983). Parent-offspring and sibling body mass index associations during and after sharing of common household environments: The Princeton school district family study. *Metabolism, 32,* 82–89.

Kingsley, R. G., & Shapiro, J. (1977). A comparison of three behavioral programs for the control of obesity in children. *Behavior Therapy, 8,* 30–36.

Kirschenbaum, D. S., Harris, E. S., & Tomarken, A. J. (1984). Effects of parental involvement in behavioral weight loss therapy for preadolescents. *Behavior Therapy, 15,* 485–500.

Klesges, R. C., Coates, T. J., Brown, G., Sturgeon–Tillisch, J., Moldenhauer-Klesges, L. M., Holzer, B., Woolfrey, J., & Vollmer, J. (1983). Parental influences on children's eating behavior and relative weight. *Journal of Applied Behavior Analysis, 16,* 371–378.

Klesges, R. C., Coates, T. J., Moldenhauer-Klesges, L. M., Holzer, B., Gustavson, J., & Barnes, J. (1984). The FATS: An observational system for assessing physical activity in children and associated parent behavior. *Behavioral Assessment, 6,* 333–345.

Klesges, R. C., Malott, J. M., Boschee, P. F., & Weber, J. M. (1986). The effects of parental influences on children's food intake, physical activity, and relative weight. *International Journal of Eating Disorders, 5,* 335–346.

Laskarzewski, P., Morrison, J. A., Khoury, P., Kelly, K., Glatfelter, L., Larsen, R., &

Glueck, C. J. (1980). Parent-child nutrient intake interrelationships in school children ages 6 to 19: The Princeton school district study. *The American Journal of Clinical Nutrition, 33,* 2350–2355.

O'Dell, S. L., Tarler-Benlolo, L., & Flynn, J. M. (1979). An instrument to measure knowledge of behavioral principles as applied to children. *Journal of Behavior Therapy and Experimental Psychiatry, 10,* 29–34.

Patterson, G. R. (1986). Performance models for antisocial boys. *American Psychologist, 41,* 432–444.

Rozin, P., Fallon, A., & Mandell, R. (1984). Family resemblance in attitudes to foods. *Developmental Psychology, 20,* 309–314.

Stunkard, A. J. (Ed.). (1980). *Obesity.* Philadelphia: Saunders.

Wooley, S. C., Wooley, O. W., & Dyrenforth, S. R. (1978). Theoretical, practical, and social issues in behavioral treatments of obesity. *Journal of Applied Behavioral Analysis, 12,* 3–25.

13

The Pittsburgh Childhood Weight Control Program: an Update

LEONARD H. EPSTEIN
University of Pittsburgh School of Medicine
Pittsburgh, Pennsylvania

I. Introduction

The purpose of this chapter is to provide a selective review of treatment development research for childhood obesity over the last decade at the University of Pittsburgh. There have been two recent reviews of this program (Epstein, 1985; Epstein, Wing and Valoski, 1985), as well as a comprehensive recent review of research on the behavioral treatment of childhood obesity (Epstein and Wing, 1987). Thus, much of the information covered in this chapter is available elsewhere. This review will provide an update on three new findings, an examination of long-term (five year) weight loss of non-participating family members, an assessment of changes in food preference after behavioral weight control, and long-term relationships between relative weight and fitness.

Children who are obese and left untreated during childhood are likely to become obese adults (Abraham, Collins and Nordsieck, 1971; Abraham and Nordsieck, 1960). In spite of recent advances in the treatment of adult obesity (Brownell and Wadden, 1986), most obese adults do not achieve and maintain ideal weight. Thus, it may be better to prevent the development of adult obesity than to wait until an obese child becomes an adult and then attempt to achieve ideal weight. Childhood obesity is not only important because it is predictive of later adult obesity. Excess weight in children is related to elevated blood pressures and elevated total cholesterol and decreased HDL cholesterol (Berenson, 1980). These risk factors track over time, so that children with elevated blood pressures or lipids may become adults with hypertension or hyperlipidemia (Clarke,

Schrott, Leaverton, Connor, and Lauer, 1978; Laskarzewski, Morrison, deGroot, Kelly, Mellies, Khoury, and Glueck, 1979).

While the relative risk of obese children becoming obese adults is increased, not all obese children will become obese adults. There are several variables which increase the relative risk of an obese child's becoming an obese adult, which may help define which children require treatment. First, the risk varies during development, with an obese six-month-old child approximately twice as likely as a non-obese six-month-old to become an obese adult (Charney, Goodman, McBride, Lyon, and Pratt, 1976), while an obese preadolescent is six times as likely as non-obese preadolescent to become an obese adult (Abraham and Nordsieck, 1960). Second, obesity runs in families (Garn and Clark, 1976), and the risk of an obese child becoming an obese adult varies with the weight of the parent (Charney et al., 1976). Third, weight status of other family members can influence the probability of a child's being obese (Garn, Bailey, Solomon, and Hopkins, 1981). Fourth, the prevalence of obesity is inversely related to family size (Jacoby, Altman, Cook and Holland, 1975). And, fifth, obesity is inversely related to socioeconomic level (Stunkard, d'Aquili, Fox, and Filion, 1972).

II. Treatment of Childhood Obesity

A. Development of Family-Based Behavioral Treatment Programs

The focus of the Pittsburgh Childhood Weight Control Program (PCWCP) is weight control by changing eating and exercise behaviors. The theoretical basis for the treatment strategies used is social learning theory (Bandura, 1969). Research has shown behavioral programs are superior to both no treatment controls (Aragona, Cassady, and Drabman, 1975; Epstein, Wing, Koeske, and Valoski, 1984; Israel, Stolmaker, Sharp, Silverman, and Simon, 1984; Kirschenbaum, Harris, and Tomarken, 1984; Weiss, 1977), and non-behavioral control treatments (Epstein, Wing, Steranchak, Dickson, and Michelson, 1980; Epstein, Wing, Penner, Kress, and Koeske, 1985; Weiss, 1977).

Our research program has emphasized a family-based approach to behavior change for two reasons. First, it is clear that familial factors are related to the development of childhood obesity. Such familial variables as food and activity availability, modeling of eating and exercise behaviors and reinforcement for eating and exercise are likely to exert important effects on childhood obesity (Epstein and Wing, 1987). Genetic factors may also be important in predicting which children will become obese adults. Genetic factors may exert independent effects on obesity, but it is likey that they interact with environmental factors to influence relative body weight (Epstein and Cluss, 1986).

In addition to the role of familial factors in the etiology of obesity, families are also important in the behavior change process. Parents are more likely to be in a position to manipulate variables that are important in the day-to-day regulation of eating and exercise behaviors than are therapists, and family-based programs are more likely than therapists to produce changes in the structure of family interactions that are important in maintaining long-term outcome than therapist-based interventions. Thus, our treatment programs, along with programs by other investigators in the area (Israel, Stolmaker, and Andrian, 1985) involve parent training in social learning.

The goals of our treatment are first to produce a significant reduction in body weight. Ideally, the change should result in the child's being less than 20% over ideal weight for height, or non-obese. Second, the treatment should teach appropriate eating and exercise habits so that the child can maintain a reduced relative weight, while getting the appropriate nutrition for growth and development. These goals must be accomplished by developing a program that is appropriate for the child's age, and developmental capabilities, and that takes into account parental influences on child habit development and change.

This program should include three components (Epstein, 1986). First, the child should be provided a diet that will produce weight loss, that is easy to adhere to, and that will promote growth. Second, the treatment should incorporate an exercise program that promotes energy expenditure, but which is also easy to adhere to. Finally, the treatment should include comprehensive training in parent management and in skill training for the older children. Behavioral training for parents and children facilitates the translation of diet and exercise information into habit change.

The main objective of this review is an overview of selected research findings in our treatment program, and not an in-depth review of our treatment procedures. The treatment procedures we use were developed initially for obese preadolescent children of obese parents, who are at particularly high risk for becoming obese adults. They have been modified and extended to younger children. As our research has evolved, the specifics of treatment have varied over time, dependent on research findings and the research questions we have asked. These procedures are detailed elsewhere, both in the individual studies reviewed and an overall review of our treatment methods and early results (Epstein, 1985). The review will cover research on behavioral, diet and exercise aspects of our treatment.

B.   Behavioral Aspects of Family-based treatment for Obese Children

The first controlled study in treatment development from our laboratory was a comparison of an early version of our behavioral treatment with a group that received equal diet and exercise information but no behavioral training (Epstein, Wing, Steranchak, Dickson, and Michelson, 1980). Since behavioral training requires more therapist time and a different type of expertise than education, this study was needed to document that behavioral treatment was important to outcome. Results showed superiority of the behavioral group over two and five months of treatment. In addition, there was a very strong relationship between parent and child weight change observed.

Our second study was designed to evaluate more carefully the effects of familial treatment variables on outcome. This study was based on two observations. Kingsley and Shapiro (1967) showed that children lost similar amounts of weight in a short-term program whether the child, parent, or parent and child was targeted, but that children did the best during follow-up if both the parent and child were targeted. In addition, we (Epstein et al., 1980) showed a strong relationship between parent and child weight loss.

The study design involved randomization of obese children with at least one obese parent to one of three groups: 1). Parent + Child targeted for weight loss; 2). Child alone targeted for weight loss; 3). Non-specific target for weight loss. The structure of the groups was similar, as was the information on diet (traffic light diet, Epstein, Wing, and Valoski, 1985) and exercise (Cooper's aerobic point system, Cooper, 1977). All families had both an obese parent and child who came to all sessions and were weighed and measured at similar intervals, but the groups differed in the behavioral contingencies for weight loss. The program involved eight weekly treatment meetings, and six meetings distributed over the next six months, with meetings bi-weekly, monthly, and then bi-monthly. Relative weight for family members was assessed at the following time periods: at the end of eight months of treatment, at 21 months for an intermediate follow-up (Epstein, Wing, Koeske, Andrasik, and Ossip, 1981), and at 60 months after beginning treatment (Epstein, Wing, Koeske and Valoski, 1987).

The major differences between the experimental and treatment groups were in the use of behavior modification between the three groups. The first behavioral technique we used was the contingency management method of teaching (Kulik, Kulik, and Cohen, 1979) to ensure that participants in the two treatment goups (I, II) knew the material that was presented to them. Information was presented in modular format, which included a self-contained lesson that presented new information and contained examples to work through, a reading quiz with answers, and a self-quiz for performance evaluation, as used by Miller (1975). In the Parent + Child group, the parent and child had to master their own respective modules, while in the Child Alone group both the parent and child had to master the child information. The information mastered was relevant to the person(s) targeted in the family. Participants in the Non-specific group were provided the same information in a more traditional lecture/ question and answer format.

The second behavior modification procedure was self-monitoring of caloric intake, exercise, and weight. In group I both the parents and child self-monitored, in group II only the child self-monitored, and in group three neither the parent nor child self-monitored. Third, parents and children in Groups I and II were trained in social learning principles. Both parents and children were taught to serve as appropriate models for eating and exercise for other family members. Also, both parents and children were taught to praise and positively support other family members for habit change. Fourth, contracting was used to promote adherence in two ways (Epstein, and Wing, 1984). First, parents in groups I and II were taught how to contract with their children, and to use incentives for weight loss. The weight loss goals were determined by the participants at each meeting, using a minimum of one pound and a maximum of three pounds. Second, contracting was used to involve differentially the parents and child in weight loss. Parents deposited $65 at the beginning of the program, with $5 returned at each treatment meeting contingent on parent *and* child weight loss in Group I, only child weight loss in Group II, or attendance in Group III. Thus, the method of promoting parent and child concurrent weight loss was to reinforce differentially parent and child weight loss across the three groups. Contracts provide a clear specification of the goals of treatment, and a consistent method for motivating the child and parent for weight loss (Epstein and Wing, 1984).

Results showed similar effects of treatment after both eight and 21 months, with all three groups showing significant changes in relative weight (Epstein et al., 1981). However, after five years, the children in Group I maintained their relative weight change (-12.7), while the children in Group II were at baseline ($+4.3$), and the children in Group III were heavier ($+8.2$). After five years 33% of the children were not obese in Group I, contrasted with 19% and 5% of the children in groups II and III. The percentage of children in Group I who were not obese was greater than that in Group III.

Participating parents showed significant differences only after eight months of treatment. At 21 and 60 months parents in the three groups did not differ. In a new analysis, we examined the effect of treatment in the three groups on non-participating obese family members (Epstein, Nudelman, and Wing, 1987). Obese siblings who were in families assigned to Group I had a significantly greater decrease in percent overweight of −7.0 after five years, while children in the other two groups combined had an increase in percent overweight of +4.1. These results parallel those of their participating siblings. The results for the non-participating parents also are similar to that for the participating parents. However, in this case, no differences across groups were shown.

Child growth over the five years of study was evaluated by first converting the actual child height into height percentiles relative to the child's age and sex. Obese children were taller than average at baseline (72nd percentile) and after five years were still above average (60th percentile) in height. While obese children are taller than their non-obese peers, they do not maintain this height difference over time, as obese adults are not taller than non-obese adults (Abraham and Johnson, 1980). Thus, they cannot be expected to remain in their same height percentile. Since the best predictor of eventual child height is parent height, height changes of the obese children were evaluated in terms of their parents' height. Children were divided into tertiles on the basis of mid-parent height (short, average, and tall at the 26th, 49th and 74th percentile, respectively). Parents had children which resembled their heights at baseline, with children of short, average, and tall parents at the 59th, 76th and 82nd percentile, respectively (p < .01). After five years of treatment the children of tall parents were at the 74th percentile, while the children of average and short parents were at the 60th and 47th percentile, respectively. Children of tall parents resemble their parents in height, while the children of average and short parents still had greater relative height than their parents.

C. Other research on parental effects.

Several other studies have investigated manipulating the role of parents in the treatment of their children. Israel et al. (1984) showed no differences at the end of nine weeks of treatment or one year of follow-up in weight loss for children with parents who self-selected (were not randomly assigned) to act as targets for weight loss versus those who chose to act as helpers. Both groups were superior to the no-treatment control at nine weeks, but the amount of weight loss at nine weeks and one year was not different. This investigative team has further found that weight loss over one year is superior for children whose parents were provided a standard weight reduction program plus two hours of parent training versus the standard weight reduction program, which included some parent training (Israel, et al. 1985). Differences in parent knowledge of behavioral principles were shown across the groups at both eight weeks and one year. Brownell, Kelman and Stunkard (1983) showed that adolescent children treated separately from their parents had superior weight loss compared to children who were seen with their parents or seen alone. However, these results were not replicated over one year of observation by Coates, Killen, and Slinkard (1982), who compared the effects of seeing the parent and child separately with seeing the child alone.

While the research by Israel (Israel et al. 1984, 1985) and Brownell (Brownell et al, 1983) showed effects of including parents in the treatment process, there are several studies (Coates et al, 1982; Kingsley and Shapiro, 1977; Kirschenbaum et al., 1984) that have shown no long-term superiority of children treated with or without their parents. The failure of parental involvement in these studies is discrepant from the other research. These results could be interpreted to suggest that children may do as well in behavior change when they control their own behavior as parents do in helping their children. However, this result was not found when programs contrasting parent control versus child self-control were studied (Epstein, Wing, Koeske and Valoski, 1986). A more likely explanation is that the results were due to differences in the content and structure of the treatment programs used or in the characteristics of subjects in these two studies. One important difference is that both of the studies failing to find effects of including the parent in treatment, treated the parent and child together, which Brownell et al (1983) have shown for adolescents is not as effective as treating both the parent and child but seeing them separately. Discrepancies within this area of research are discussed in more depth by Epstein and Wing (1987).

A second area of research was the comparison of parent control versus child self-control. The previous two studies discussed were based on parent manipulation of the important familial variables that may influence child eating and activity. However, there are several reasons to attempt to develop programs that may promote child self-control of eating and exercise. First, Cohen, Gelfand, Dodd, Jensen and Turner (1980) showed that child self-control was related to success in long-term weight control. In addition, self-control is a concept that is conceptually related to success in weight control. For this reason one of the purposes of the study by Epstein, Wing, Koeske, and Valoski (1986) was to compare a child self-managed (SC) to parent managed (PM) treatment. The child self-control procedures were based on methods recommended by O'Leary and Dubey (1979). Research in this area suggests that self-control in children is best accomplished when control of the relevant goal setting and reinforcement are first developed under the control of an external change agent (parent), and then faded to the child. Examination of the effects of these procedures (PM vs. SC) over a five-year period showed no differences between these two treatment strategies. Thus, child self-control may be as good as parent control, but not better than parent control.

However, this is the only study on this important component of childhood weight control, and the issue should not be considered closed. There is continuing interest in child development on new methods of promoting child self-control (Kendall and Finch, 1979) that may prove to be important. In addition, improvements in certain program components, such as more gradual fading from parent to child control, better specification of the goal behaviors and the relationship between goal behavior and reinforcement and improved control over goal setting and response-reinforcer contingency development may have resulted in child self-control's being superior to parent control. Additional research on this important topic is needed.

D.   Modification of eating behavior

1. *Diet.*   The traffic light diet was designed to promote weight loss, to provide adequate calories and nutrients for growth and development, and to be easy to adhere to. The diet divides foods into eleven categories, with the foods in each category then separated into three color groups: green, yellow, and red. These colors correspond to the colors of a traffic light, and signify GO (Green), eat as much as you like; approach with CAUTION (Yellow), eat in moderate amounts; and STOP (Red), do not eat. Examples of foods in the three categories are presented in Table 1.

Green foods are those foods that contain less than 20 calories per average serving, and are contained only in the vegetable and free foods

Table I

Examples of Foods in the Traffic-Light Diet

Food Group	Green	Yellow	Red
Vegetables	Asparagus	Corn	Scalloped Potatoes
Fruits	Lemon juice	Apple	Fruit in heavy syrup
High protein		Baked fish	Fried fish
Milk & Dairy		Skim Milk	Whole Milk
Grains		Bagel	Donut
Other	Herbs & Spices	Italian dressing	Candy
Combined Items		Chop Suey	Lasagna

categories. Yellow foods are foods that are within 20 calories per average serving of the caloric value of the average food within that food group. Yellow foods are items from the basic four food groups which a child should eat in recommended amounts in order to obtain adequate nutrition. Red foods are foods that exceed the caloric value of a yellow food, thereby lowering the nutrient density of the food. In addition, red foods include any food that is made to resemble a red food, as low calorie lasagna, which might not be a red food in terms of calories, but is labeled a red food because persons will not break the habit of eating lasagna if they often substitute low for high calorie lasagna. This is a rule designed to prevent the participant's generalizing the preference for the imitation food to the higher calorie food that served as the model. Finally, a food becomes a red food when a combined dish or casserole includes red food components, or is over 300 calories per serving. This rule is designed to teach parents and children to limit portion sizes, and eat a wide variety of foods. Participants were limited to four red foods per week.

In addition to using the diet to improve food selection by decreasing caloric cost of foods without decreasing nutrient intake, the diet also emphasizes the child's obtaining a balance of the major food groups while caloric intake is being decreased. As part of the habit book that the child uses to record food intake, the number of servings from each of the basic four food groups are recorded, and parents are instructed to praise children for eating the appropriate number of servings from each food group. Our initial caloric intake level was 1200 calories for boys, girls and mothers; men greater than 200 pounds were given a 1500 calorie limit. These levels have been reduced and standardized in our three programs. Children 1–5, 5–8, and 8 and older have different caloric requirements and different balance of the four food groups that are based on the recommended daily allowances for essential nutrients (Food and Nutrition Board, 1980). The number of servings of foods along with the portion size within each food group are shown in Table 2. The nutrient intakes of children in our programs is available elsewhere (Epstein, Wing, and Valoski, 1985).

2. *Food preference.*   Behavioral treatment programs are designed to modify eating behavior, as well as to affect reductions in caloric intake and intake of a balanced diet. However, there is very little research designed to document methods of changing eating. We have shown that changes in intake of high calorie foods are related to intermediate (Epstein et al, 1981) and long term (Epstein et al, 1987) weight loss in our standard program. While decrease in intake of high calorie foods is important to treatment success, most dieters return to old eating habits and do not maintain their weight loss. One reason for these failures may

Table II

Nutritional Balance of the Diet for Children of Different Ages

Food Groups	Servings	1–3	4–6	Age 7–10	11–14	Adult
Dairy	2–5	1/2C	1/2C	3/4C	1C	1C
Skim milk						
Grain	at least 4					
Bread		1/2Sl	1/2–3/4Sl	3/4–1Sl	1Sl	1Sl
Cereal/Pasta &						
Starchy						
Vegetables		1/4–1/3C	1/3–1/2C	3/4C	1C	1C
Fruits &	at least 4					
Vegetables						
Citrus	1	1/4C	1/3C	1/2C	1/2C	1/2C
Leafy green or	1	3T	1/4C	1/3C	1/2C	1/2C
dark orange						
Vegetable						
Other fruit or	2–3	3T	1/4C	1/3C	1/2C	1/2C
vegetable						
Protein Group	2					
Egg	1 every other day	1 med	1 med	1 med	1 med	1 med
Lean Meat,	1	1oz	2oz	3oz	3oz	3oz
Fish, Poultry						
Polyunsaturated	total	1	3	3	4.5	4.5
Oil	tsp/day					
Calories*		900–1300	900–1300	900–1200	900–1200	female 900–1200 male 900–1500

* Calorie limits were obtained for a 1–5 year old child by subtracting 200 calories from their normal intake, with the exception that an upper limit of 1300 and a lower limit of 900 was set.

Abbreviations   Sl = slice, C = cup, T = tablespoon, tsp = teaspoon.

be the failure to attend to food preferences. Increasing the preference of obese children for lower calorie foods could be important in ensuring that children will make choices of low calorie versus high calorie foods when given availability of either type.

Birch, Zimmerman and Hind (1980) have shown that novel foods that are used to reinforce other behaviors, or foods that are paired with parental attention will show increases in their preference. On the basis of this finding, we attempted to use novel low calorie foods to reinforce adherence to the program for one group, with the goal of increasing preference for these foods (Epstein, Wing, Valoski, and Penner, 1987). This group was compared to another group that increased their intake of the novel foods, but independent of behavior. Previous research has also shown that increased familiarity can result in increases in preference. However, assessment of preference by rank order methods at the end of treatment and after six months was not related to any changes in food preference.

Additional research, using new methods of measuring and modifying food preference, is needed to provide technologies for both short and long term modification of food preferences. One possible approach may be to increase the preference for foods by classical conditioning; Zellner, Rozin, Aron, and Kulish (1983) have shown that pairing a novel food with a sweet taste can result in increased preference for that food without the sweetness. In addition, Rolls, Rolls and Rowe (1982) have shown that variety of foods is related to preference, with a positive relationship between the number of foods available and the preference for those foods. Reduction in the number of foods eaten during a diet may decrease the preference and appetite for those foods, resulting in less chance for overeating and breaking the rules of the diet.

E.   Exercise and Childhood Weight Loss

Our exercise research has focused on two types of exercise programs, structured (programmed) aerobic exercise, or life-style exercise programs that can be differentiated for use in the treatment of obesity (Brownell and Stunkard, 1980; Epstein, Koeske, and Wing, 1984). Other types of exercise programs that do not emphasize caloric expenditure, as body shaping or toning, are not as relevant to changes in energy balance and thus are probably less important in weight loss than those that increase caloric expenditure (Brownell and Stunkard, 1980).

We have completed four studies which assess the role of exercise in the treatment of childhood obesity. The first study in this series (Epstein, Wing, Koeske, Ossip and Beck, 1982) assessed isocaloric life-style and programmed aerobic exercise crossed with diet/no diet. The results showed equal effects of life-style and aerobic exercise during the initial two-month treatment, which was expected since the two exercise programs were isocaloric. In addition, the aerobic program showed greater fitness effects, also expected, since the aerobic exercise was of greater intensity. By six months, and continuing to 17 months, the life-style exercise was superior to the programmed aerobic exercise. Aerobic versus life-style exercise was compared in a second study (Epstein, Wing, Koeske and Valoski, 1985) with a different methodology. The study compared three groups that each had diet, but differed in the type of exercise. Isocaloric aerobic and life-style exercises were compared to a plausible placebo exercise, calisthenics, which was similar in the amount of exercise time required goal setting and feedback, but which involved considerably less caloric expenditure. The inclusion of a control group provided a realistic, low expenditure exercise program, which is important to control for many of the non-specific components of exercise that may influence weight that are not a function of caloric expenditure (Epstein and Wing, 1980). The results of this study showed no differences in relative weight change at 12 months; however at 24 months the life-style group (−18.0%) had lost significantly more than the programmed aerobic (−6.8%) or the calisthenics (−7.2%). The most probable mechanism for the long-term differences would be better adherence in life-style than the aerobic group, though exercise adherence was not measured over time.

In two additional studies we evaluated the effects of diet plus exercise versus diet alone. Since exercise increases caloric expenditure, it was expected that adding exercise would increase weight loss. In the first of these two studies we randomized obese parents and children to one of three groups: diet + life-style exercise, diet, and no treatment control (Epstein, Wing, Koeske, and Valoski, 1984). The diet group was provided a very low expenditure stretching exercise program. Results showed the expected effects for the parents, that diet plus exercise was superior to diet alone at six and twelve months, but there were no differences observed for the children.

We hypothesized that the failure to observe effects for children was due to poor adherence to exercise. To reduce adherence problems children exercised with the experimenters in a standardized treatment program. Children were randomized to a standard diet treatment program, or a diet program plus a six-week, three-day per week summer camp (Epstein, Wing, Penner, Kress, and Kalsker, 1985). After twelve months, the diet plus exercise group showed the expected superiority (−25.4% overweight) compared to the control group (−18.7% overweight). These results suggest that adherence is playing a role in the failure to show differential effectiveness of diet plus exercise versus diet alone.

These exercise results suggest that life-style exercise is superior for the treatment of childhood obesity than more programmed, higher intensity aerobic exercise. However, much additional research in this area is needed. First, eating and exercise behavior has not been measured during follow-up periods actually documenting that children adhere better to life-style exercise compared to aerobic exercise. The differences may be in terms of different eating in the two groups, or a combination of differences in eating and exercising. Second, many investigators would prefer aerobic exercise to isocaloric life-style exercise, as the aerobic exercise would result in better fitness improvement. Thus, there is the important need for additional research on behavioral methods for improving adherence to aerobic exercise in obese children. Given the general problems of adherence to exercise (Martin and Dubbert, 1982), these methods could be useful for children with problems other than obesity.

1. *Fitness improvement with weight loss.* We have examined the relationship between changes in weight or relative weight and fitness in obese children treated across several programs that included fitness assessment. The first analysis compared the degree of heart rate change to a standardized workload using the Montoye Step Test over a six month period. Most children showed a decrease in relative weight over this interval, and they were divided into three groups based on the amount of change in relative weight and their final relative weight. High success children showed greater heart rate change than children in the other two groups (Epstein, Koeske, Zidansek, and Wing, 1983).

We recently have completed an analysis of changes in relative weight and fitness over five years. Multivariate regression analysis predicting the fitness change over five years showed the influence of two variables: initial fitness level and maintenance of weight loss after six months of treatment to the five-year follow-up. Children who were the least fit, and who had the largest long-term changes in relative weight showed the largest improvements in fitness.

E.   The Influence of Parent Weight on Child Weight Loss

One important factor that is related to the risk of an obese child becoming an obese adult is parent weight. Parent weight may exert effects on child outcome by a variety of behavioral or genetic factors (Epstein and Cluss, 1986). Whatever the mechanism, it could be predicted that obese children with obese parents will not be as successful in weight control as obese children with non-obese parents. We evaluated the effect of parental weight [two thin (TP) versus at least one obese (HP)] on child relative weight change over three (Epstein, Wing, Koeske, and Valoski, 1986) and five year (Epstein, Wing, Valoski and Gooding, 1987) periods. The five-year follow-up data show that obese children with thin or obese parents show similar changes in relative weight after six months, with children with non-obese parents maintaining the changes from six−twelve months, while obese children with obese parents regressed towards baseline levels. Children with both obese or thin parents showed increases in relative weight over time, but the differences observed at one year were maintained from one to five years. These results suggest that obese children of obese parents are both more likely to become obese adults than obese children of thin parents (Charney et al., 1976), and may not benefit as much from treatment as obese children of thin parents. This differential effect of weight loss by parent weight may account for variability often observed in treatment results across studies. It is possible that the differences observed at five years simply reflect natural developmental changes that would have occurred for obese offspring of obese or non-obese parents. Treatment may have accelerated the shift of obese children with obese parents toward non-obese status.

G.   Obesity Treatment for Younger children

The previous research we have presented from our laboratory has been with eight–twelve-year-old children. Due to the increased risk with child age, it may be possible to extend our program to younger children and prevent obesity earlier. We have shown a parent-managed, family-based treatment program was superior to a health education control group for five–eight-year-old girls (Epstein, Wing, Woodall, Penner, Kress, and Koeske, 1985). In addition, we have shown significant relative weight changes that have been maintained over two years in a sample of 17 obese toddlers treated in a program that included diet, exercise, and parent management. The magnitude of change for these young children was very similar to the amount of change observed for the older children. In addition, no changes in the height percentile of these children was observed over the treatment (Epstein, Valoski, Koeske, and Wing, 1986).

H.   Areas for future research.

The research we have completed on childhood obesity is promising, but we are only in the initial stages of development of powerful treatments that will allow obese children to become non-obese children and then non-obese adults. With this goal in mind, we have outlined two broad areas of research that we plan to focus on in the future. The first area is related to the effects of family-based treatment we have observed on non-treated siblings (Epstein, Nudelman, and Wing, 1987). These changes suggest that treatment effects generalize to other children in the family. Given that obesity runs in families, and many families have more than one obese child, understanding the mechanisms for the generalization of treatment effects across siblings may improve the treatment effectiveness over several obese family members. Likewise, understanding the mechanisms that influence weight loss in siblings may be useful for improving treatment efforts for the targeted child.

Second, we need to complete the long-term follow-up for children treated in each of our treatment studies to better understand variables that are important to long-term treatment effectiveness. It has often been observed that variables important in the acquisition of a habit are different from those that maintain the new behavior. For this reason, the effectiveness of treatments often decreases over time. However, since the goal of treatment is long-term weight regulation, it is imperative that treatments focus on variables that persist in regulating weight during the development of the child.

III. Summary

There are several points that can be made based on the research reviewed.

1). Behavioral treatment procedures are effective in treating childhood obesity. Changes in relative weight have been observed for periods up to five years.

2). The inclusion of parents in the treatment process is important for treatment success. Results may be improved by targeting and reinforcing weight and habit change for both parents and children versus children alone. In addition, it may be best to see the parent and child separately in treatment meetings, rather than together.

3). Life-style exercise programs may be associated with better weight loss than aerobic exercise programs.

4). Adherence to exercise is likely to be a problem with obese children, and the choice or design of an exercise program should take these adherence problems into account.

5). The family-based treatment for childhood obesity developed for pre-adolescent children can be adapted successfully for the treatment of younger children.

In summary, a growing body of research has emerged which has identified important risk factors which place a child at an increased risk of becoming an obese adult. Treatments have been developed and refined that are associated with both significant and long-lasting effects on childhood weight status. Additional research on the development of treatment methods is needed to prevent and treat childhood obesity.

Acknowledgments

The preparation of this manuscript, and the research reported, were supported in part by Grants HD19532 and HD20829 from the National Institute of Child Health and Human Development.

References

Aragona, J., Cassady, J., & Drabman, R. S. (1975). Treating overweight children through parental training and contingency contracting. *Journal of Applied Behavior Analysis, 8*, 269–278.

Abraham, S., Collins, G., & Nordsieck, M. (1971). Relationship of childhood weight status to morbidity in adults. *Public Health Reports, 85*, 273–284.

Abraham, S., & Johnson, C. L. (1980). Prevalence of severe obesity in the United States. *American Journal of Clinical Nutrition, 33*, 364–369.

Abraham, S., & Nordsieck, M. (1960). Relationship of excess weight in children and adults. *Public Health Reports, 75*, 263–273.

Bandura, A. (1969). *Principles of Behavior Modification*. New York: Holt, Rinehart & Winston.

Berenson, G. S. (1980). *Cardiovascular Risk Factors in Children: The Early Natural History of Atherosclerosis and Essential Hypertension*. New York: Oxford University Press.

Birch, L. L., Zimmerman, S. I., & Hind, H. (1980). The influence of social affective context on the formation of children's food preferences. *Child Development, 51*, 856–861.

Brownell, K. D., Kelman, S. H., & Stunkard, A. J. (1983). Treatment of obese children with and without their mothers: Changes in weight and blood pressure. *Pediatrics, 71*, 515–523.

Brownell, K. D., & Stunkard, A. J. (1980). Physical activity in the development and control of obesity. In A. J. Stunkard (Ed.), *Obesity* (pp. 300–324). Saunders: Philadelphia.

Brownell, K. D., & Wadden, T. A. (1986). Behavior therapy for obesity: Modern approaches and better results. In K. D. Brownell & J. P. Foreyt (Eds.), *Handbook of Eating Disorders* (pp. 180–197). New York: Basic Books.

Charney, E., Goodman, H. C., McBride, M., Lyon, B., & Pratt, R. (1976). Childhood antecedents of adult obesity. Do chubby infants become obese adults? *New England Journal of Medicine, 295*, 6–9.

Clarke, W. R., Schrott, H. G., Leaverton, P. E., Connor, W. E., & Lauer, R. M. (1978). Tracking of blood lipids and blood pressures in school age children: The Muscatine study. *Circulation, 58*, 626–634.

Coates, T. J., Killen, J. D., & Slinkard, L. A. (1982). Parent participation in a treatment program for overweight adolescents. *International Journal of Eating Disorders, 1*, 37–48.

Cohen, E. A., Gelfand, D. M., Dodd, D. K., Jensen, J., & Turner, C. (1980). Self-control practices associated with weight loss maintenance in children and adolescents. *Behavior Therapy, 11*, 26–37.

Cooper, K. H. (1977). *The Aerobics Way*. New York: M. Evans.

Epstein, L. H. (1985). Family-based treatment for pre-adolescent obesity. In M. L. Wolraich & D. Routh (Eds.), *Advances in Developmental and Behavioral Pediatrics*. Greenwich, CT: Jai Press. pp. 1–39.

Epstein, L. H. (1986). Treatment of childhood obesity. In K. D. Brownell & J. P. Foreyt (Eds.), *Handbook of Eating Disorders* (pp. 159–179). New York: Basic Books.

Epstein, L. H., & Cluss, P. A. (1986). Behavioral genetics of childhood obesity. *Behavior Therapy, 17*, 324–334.

Epstein, L. H., Koeske, R., & Wing, R. R. (1984). Adherence to exercise in obese children. *Journal of Cardiac Rehabilitation, 4*, 185–195.

Epstein, L. H., Koeske, R., Zidansek, J., & Wing, R. R. (1983). Effects of weight loss on fitness in obese children. *American Journal of Diseases of Children, 137*, 654–657.

Epstein, L. H., Nudelman, S., & Wing, R. R. (1987). Long term effects of famiy-based treatment on nontreated family members. *Behavior Therapy, 12*, 147–152.

Epstein, L. H., Valoski, A., Koeske, R., & Wing, R. R. (1986). Behavioral weight control in obese young children. *Journal of the American Dietetic Association, 86,* 481−484.

Epstein, L. H., & Wing, R. R. (1980). Aerobic exercise and weight. *Addictive Behaviors, 5,* 371−388.

Epstein, L. H. & Wing, R. R. (1984). Behavioral contracting: Health behaviors. In C. M. Franks (Ed.), *New Directions in Behavior Therapy: From Research to Clinical Application* (pp. 409−450.). New York: Haworth Press.

Epstein, L. H., & Wing, R. R. (1987). Behavioral treatment of childhood obesity. *Psychological Bulletin, 101,* 331−342.

Epstein, L. H., Wing, R. R., Koeske, R., Andrasik, F., & Ossip, D. J. (1981). Child and parent weight loss in family-based behavioral modification programs. *Journal of Consulting and Clinical Psychology, 49,* 674−685.

Epstein, L. H., Wing, R. R., Koeske, R., Ossip, D. J., & Beck, S. (1982). A comparison of life-style change and programmed aerobic exercise on weight and fitness changes in obese children. *Behavior Therapy, 13,* 651−665.

Epstein, L. H., Wing, R. R., Koeske, R., & Valoski, A. (1984). The effects of diet plus exercise on weight change in parents and children. *Journal of Consulting and Clinical Psychology, 52,* 429−437.

Epstein, L. H., Wing, R. R., Koeske, R., & Valoski, A. (1985). A comparison of life-style exercise, aerobic exercise, and calisthenics on weight loss in obese children. *Behavior Therapy, 16,* 345−356.

Epstein, L. H., Wing, R. R., Koeske, R., & Valoski, A. (1986). The effects of parental weight on child weight loss. *Journal of Consulting and Clinial Psychology, 54,* 400−401.

Epstein, L. H., Wing, R. R., Koeske, R., & Valoski, A. (1987). Long-term efects of family-based treatment of childhood obesity. *Journal of Consulting and Clinical Psychology, 55,* 91−95.

Epstein, L. H., Wing, R. R., Penner, B., Kress M. J., & Koeske, R. (1985). The effect of diet and controlled exercise on weight loss in obese children. *Journal of Pediatrics, 107,* 358−361.

Epstein, L. H., Wing, R. R., Steranchak, L., Dickson, B., & Michelson, J. (1980). Comparison of family-based behavior modification and nutrition education for childhood obesity. *Journal of Pediatric Psychology, 5,* 25−36.

Epstein, L. H., Wing, R. R., & Valoski, A. (1985). Childhood Obesity. *Pediatric Clinics of North America, 32,* 363−379.

Epstein, L. H., Wing, R. R., Valoski, A., & Gooding, W. (1987). Long-term effects of parent weight on child weight loss. *Behavior Therapy, 18,* 219−226.

Epstein, L. H., Wing, R. R., Valoski, A, & Penner, B. C. (1987). Stability of food preferences in 8−12 year old children and their parents during weight control. *Behavior Modification, 11,* 87−101.

Epstein, L. H., Wing, R. R., Woodall, K., Penner, B. C., Kress, M. J., & Koeske, R. (1985). Effects of family-based behavioral treatment on obese 5−8-year-old children. *Behavior Therapy, 16,* 205−212.

Food and Nutrition Board. (1980). *Recommended Dietary Allowances: 9th Edition.* Washington, D.C.: National Academy of Sciences.

Garn, S. M., Bailey, S. M., Solomon, M. A., & Hopkins, P. J. (1981). Effect of remaining family members on fatness prediction. *American Journal of Clinical Nutrition, 34,* 148−153.

Garn, S. M., & Clark, D. C. (1976). Trends in fatness and the origins of obesity. *Pediatrics, 57,* 443−456.

Israel, A. C., Stolmaker, L., & Andrian, C. A. G. (1985). The effects of training parents in general child management skills on a behavioral weight loss program for children. *Behavior Therapy, 16,* 169−180.

Israel, A. C., Stolmaker, L., Sharp, J. P., Silverman, W. K., & Simon, L. G. (1984). An evaluation of two methods of parental involvement in treating obese children. *Behavior Therapy, 15*, 266–272.

Jacoby, A., Altman, D. G., Cook, J., & Holland, W. W. (1975). Influence of some social and environmental factors on the nutrient intake and nutritional status of schoolchildren. *British Journal of Preventive Social Medicine, 29*, 116–120.

Kendall, P. C., & Finch, A. J. (1979). Developing nonimpulsive behavior in children: Cognitive-Behavioral Strategies for Self-Control. In P. C. Kendall & S. D. Hollon (Eds.), *Cognitive-Behavioral Interventions: Theory, Research, and Procedures (pp. 37–80)*. New York: Academic Press.

Kingsley, R. G., & Shapiro, J. (1977). A comparison of three behavioral programs for the control of obesity in children. *Behavior Therapy, 8*, 30–36.

Kirschenbaum, D. S., Harris, E. S., & Tomarken, A. J. (1984). Effects of parental involvement in behavioral weight loss therapy for preadolescents. *Behavior Therapy, 15*, 485–500.

Kulik, J. A., Kulik, C. C., & Cohen, P. A. (1979). A meta-analysis of outcome studies of Keller's personalized system of instruction. *American Psychologist, 34*, 307-318.

Laskarzewski, P., Morrison, J. A., deGroot, I., Kelly, K. A., Mellies, M. J., Khoury, P., & Glueck, C. J. (1979). Lipid and lipoprotein tracking in 108 children over 4-year period. *Pediatrics, 64*, 584–591.

Martin, J. E., & Dubbert, P. M. (1982). Exercise applications and promotion in behavioral medicine: Current status and future directions. *Journal of Consulting and Clinical Psychology, 50*, 1004–1017.

Miller, L. K. (1975). *Principles of Everyday Behavior Analysis*. Monterey, CA: Brooks/Cole.

O'Leary, S. G., & Dubey, D. R. (1979). Application of self-control procedures by children: A review. *Journal of Applied Behavior Analysis, 12*, 449–466.

Rolls, B. J., Rolls, E. T., & Rowe, E. A. (1982). The influence of variety on human selection and intake. In L. M. Barker (Ed.) *The Psychobiology of Human Food Selection* (pp. 101–122). Westport, CT: AVI.

Stunkard, A., d'Aquili, E., Fox, S., & Filion, D. L. (1972). Influence of social class on obesity and thinness in children. *Journal of the American Medical Association, 221*, 579–584.

Weiss, A. R. (1977). A behavioral approach to the treatment of adolescent obesity. *Behavior Therapy, 8*, 720–726.

Zellner, D. A., Rozin, P., Aron, M., & Kulish, C. Conditioned enhancement of human's liking for flavor by pairing with sweetness. (1983). *Learning and Motivation, 11*, 338–350.

Index